Blonde Beautiful Blonde

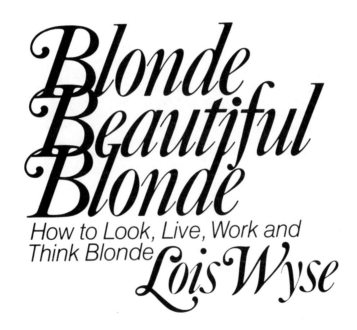

Blonde Beautiful Blonde

How to Look, Live, Work and
Think Blonde

Lois Wyse

M. Evans and Company, Inc.

New York

Thanks are due to the following for material included in this book:

Ronald Alter of Ron's Now & Then for photographs pp. x, 5, 20-24. *Clairol, Inc.* for photographs pp. 35, 113, 168, 172-175. *Columbia Pictures* for photograph p. 51 (Meryl Streep); photograph by Henry Wolfe. *Cosmopolitan* Magazine for photograph p. 121 (Christie Brinkley); photograph by Francesco Scavullo. *Culver Pictures* for photograph p. 43 (Grace Kelly). *The Hearst Corporation* for: color photographs following p. 86, copyright © 1976, 1978, 1979, 1980 by The Hearst Corporation; p. 26 (Farah Fawcett), copyright © 1978 by The Hearst Corporation, photograph by Sherman Weisburd; p. 36 (Cheryl Ladd), copyright © 1979 by The Hearst Corporation, photograph by Charles Bush. *The Metropolitan Museum of Art* for illustrations pp. 18-19; all rights reserved. *Orion Pictures/Warner Brothers* for photograph p. 84 (Bo Derek). *Random House* for exercises pp. 120-121 from *Miss Craig's 21-Day Shape-Up Program* by Marjorie Craig; copyright © 1968; reprinted by permission of Random House, Inc. *Sygma* for photograph p. 68 (Catherine Deneuve). *Maje Waldo* for photograph p. 161 (Suzan Couch). *Warner Brothers* for photograph p. 123 (Dina Merrill).

Library of Congress Cataloging in Publication Data

Wyse, Lois.
    Blonde beautiful blonde.
    1. Beauty, Personal. 2. Women—Health and
hygiene. 3. Cosmetics. I. Title.
RA778.W97   646.7   80-10551
ISBN 0-87131-311-1

Copyright © 1980 by Lois Wyse
Illustrations © 1980 by M. Evans and Company, Inc.

M. Evans and Company, Inc.
216 East 49 Street
New York, New York 10017

Design by Richard Voehl

Manufactured in the United States of America

9 8 7 6 5 4 3 2 1

For every woman
who is blonde at heart.

Contents

(continued)

(continued)

Living the Blonde Life 114

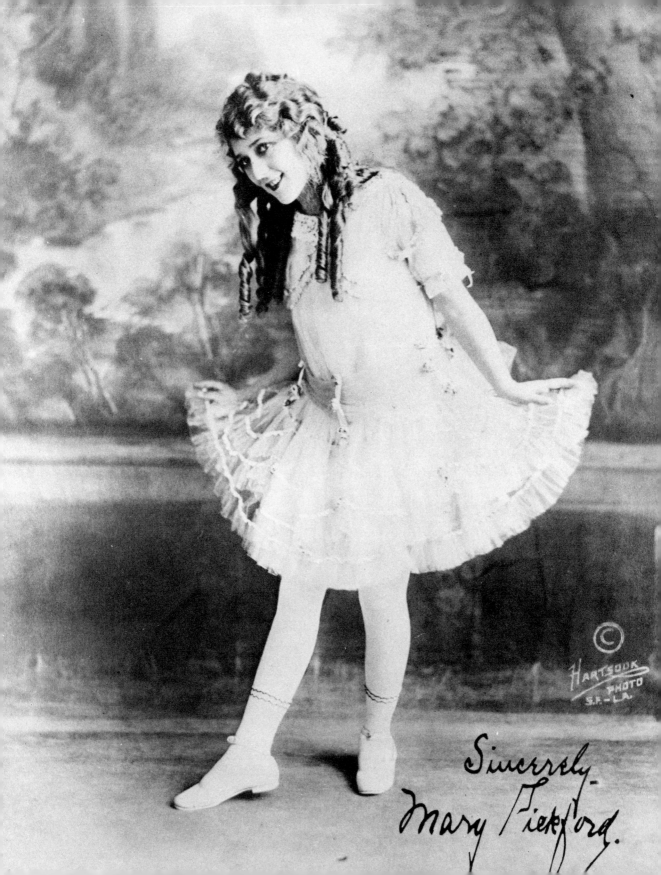

Sincerely,
Mary Pickford.

Introduction

Elizabeth Taylor shouldn't do it.

Joan Crawford did it once and hated it.

Still there are thousands of ordinary women who every day take a deep breath and make an extraordinary commitment to The Blonde Life. I'm one of them.

And unlike jogging, exercise and diet enthusiasts, I don't think everyone should do what I did. But I do think every woman—absolutely every woman who thinks life could be better than it is—should consider it.

That's what this book is about: going blonde, being blonde, staying blonde. This book is about blonde and shapely, blonde and healthy, blonde and beautiful— but above all blonde.

Is blonde worth it?

Is it worth the time, effort and money?

Is it worth the effect it will have on the people who know you—not to mention those who love you?

Only you can decide.

Going blonde is easier done than said.

Deciding takes years. Doing is a matter of hours. The process of reviving childhood blondeness (a born-again blonde) or changing to blonde takes less time than flying from New York to Los Angeles, is cheaper than a winter coat and more exciting than losing ten pounds.

Yet if she has spent thirty years as a would-be blonde, nothing in the world makes a woman feel more in command of herself than looking in the mirror and seeing her face surrounded by blonde hair.

As one thirtyish woman said, "All my life I had mousy brown hair. It was boring brown, and one day I realized I felt as boring as my hair. Then I went blonde. Now when I walk down the street people say, 'Hi, Blondie.' All those other years nobody ever stopped to say, 'Hi, Brownie.' "

Blonde is more than a hair color. It's a way of dressing and wearing makeup. It's the movement and the shape of your body, the background look of your life.

Being blonde can change the way you live.

Having blonde hair is only part of being blonde. You also have to have the right kind of body, buoyancy, makeup, wardrobe and background to really enjoy blondeness.

You have to get the answers to questions most blondes want to ask, but don't know how to get answered.

For instance . . .

Should you wear turquoise? (Probably not.)

Is pink one of the best colors to paint your living room? (Absolutely.)

Can you dye your poodle to match your hair? (Don't try.)

Those are the kinds of questions you can't get answered in one place. I know because I looked for answers in books, and I couldn't find them.

So I went to hundreds of experts, asked a lot of questions and had an extraordinary amount of help from people in all walks of life: social scientists, researchers, beauticians, designers, executives. They are credited throughout the book.

I am particularly grateful to Clairol because I'm convinced that no book on blonding can be written without the full help and guidance of the remarkable company that turned the American blonde from a platinum caricature into a dazzling, healthy-looking woman.

So my thanks to Bruce S. Gelb, executive vice president of Bristol-Myers; Donald J. Shea, president of Clairol; Dr. John Menkart, senior vice president-technology; Mary Grace Hannon, director-market planning and research; Helen Kaufmann, senior associate director-market planning and research; Cathi Hunt, director-consumer satisfaction; Gillian Hee, consumer relations manager; Phyllis Klein, director of publicity; Vern Silberman, director of product performance; the late Sheldon Levison.

In addition I want to express my appreciation to Richard Voehl, who designed the book; Katherine Wyse, who supervised research; to Sandra J. Albert and Mary Ann Shea who assisted. Among the most helpful was a panel of experts I consulted to help develop the total Beautiful Blonde life style. These people are Victor Vito, hair; Sara McBandy, makeup; Annelle Warwick, interior design; Emily Cho and Giorgio Sant'Angelo, fashion; Harold Frishman, stylist and partner HBA furs; Eva Pusta, fashion editor, jewelry; Lois L. Lindauer, nutrition. Special thanks to my special secretary, Karen Asmanis.

And to Linda C. Exman, the perceptive editor who first said to me, "Why don't you do a really comprehensive book about what it's like to be blonde?"

Well, Linda, this is what it's like.

The Importance of Being Blonde

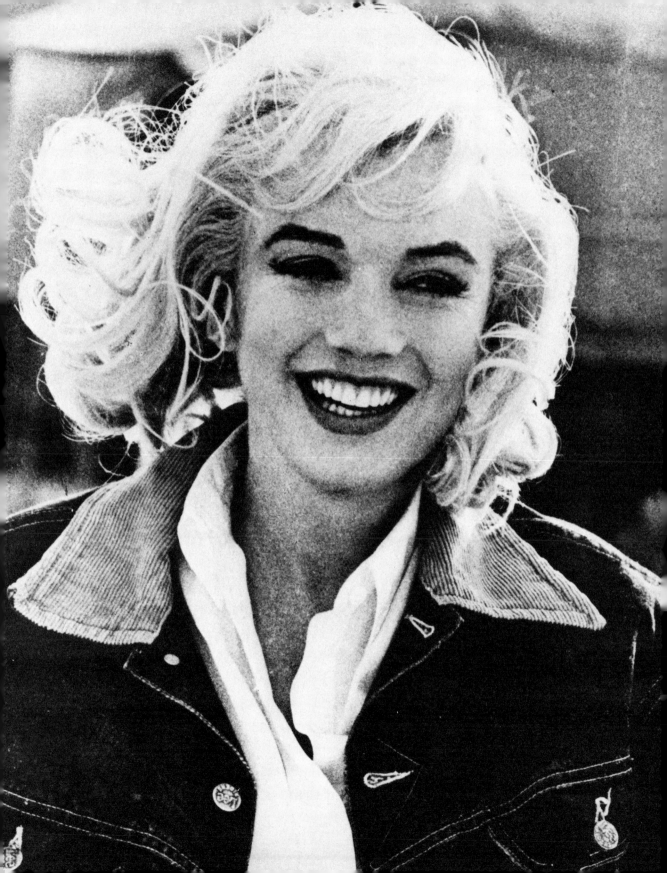

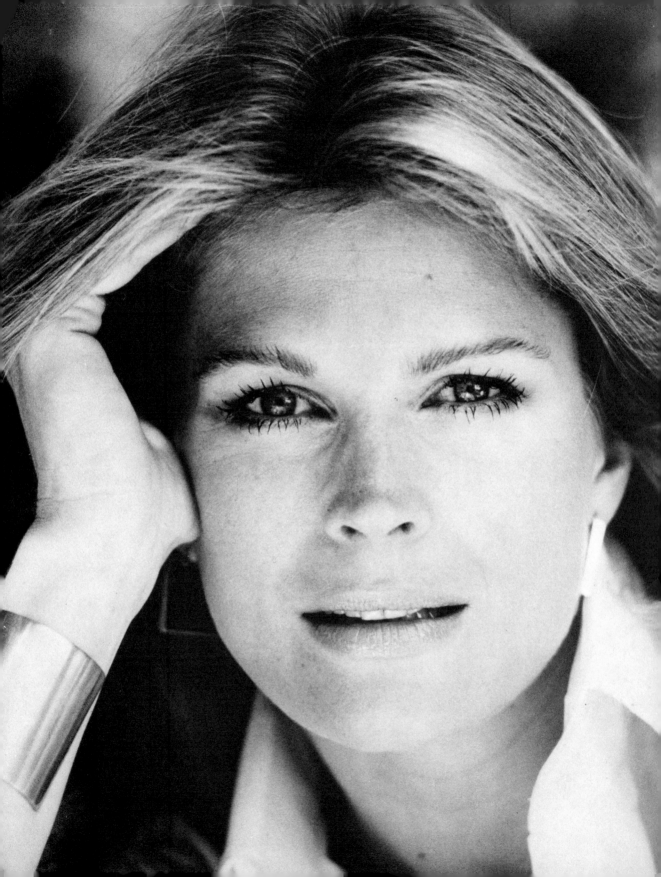

The Blonde State of Mind

"The trouble is that the blonde image is too horizontal for most vertical thinkers."

Barbaralee Diamonstein

Candice Bergen: reflecting the blonde state of mind

The Blonde Myth

The preoccupation with blondes isn't an American phenomenon. Blondes have a special cachet all over the world.

Orientals have always thought of fair-haired women as awesome and godlike.

Blonde meant divinity and aristocracy to the people of Egypt, Greece and Rome.

And back in the Middle Ages poets heralded the blonde as "the ideal woman."

Our reverence for blondes begins early in life.

Angels, a classic representation of purity and goodness, are always blonde.Witches, on the other hand, are dark.

All through mythology we learn that good is light; evil, black.

A child's first encounter with literature firmly plants The Blonde Myth. Says Dr. Joyce Brothers, "Ask a kindergarten boy to draw a beautiful lady. He'll immediately put blonde hair on her. All fairy princesses and everyone who is desirable in fairy tales is a blonde. Snow White is the only exception I can think of."

For little girls the myth of blonde and blue-eyed is reinforced in the toy department. As recently as 1977, despite the pressure from ethnic groups, almost all dolls were blonde and blue-eyed. A spokesman for Mattel Toy Makers admitted, "A doll can have any color hair as long as it's blonde."

And so it continues throughout the formative years.

High school girls for three generations have been raised with the dream of the golden-haired cheerleader who is voted Homecoming Queen and goes to the Prom with the football captain.

Who can guess how many gallons of lemon juice

have been squeezed over how many millions of dish-water-blonde heads in an effort to make a teenage girl's hair look golden?

How many young girls have sweated and stewed in the midday sun waiting for the sunshine to turn their drab brown hair something close to blonde?

And how many girls have sobbed over a botched-up color job administered by a teenage friend?

Why all the concentration on blonde?

Because The Blonde Myth means more to a woman than being beautiful. It is an embodiment of romantic dreams. And despite liberation, equal pay for equal work and the independent spirit, there are still women who are in love with romance.

The Psychoanalytic View

Dr. Theodore Isaac Rubin, the psychiatrist, says, "Of course women like to be blonde, and men like blondes. It's more American, cleaner, more Anglo-Saxon."

In random interviewing for this book I found that one-time brown- or dark-haired women who became blonde could pinpoint the day they became blonde.

A doctor said, "I became blonde the day I divorced my first husband. He always hated blonde hair. I always wanted it."

An editor changed her hair color the day after her father died.

In neither case was the woman trying to deny her identity—merely to change it to dramatize a change in her life.

Dr. Alexandra Symonds, a psychiatrist with the Karen Horney Clinic, says, "By the time a woman has become an adult she's absorbed the culture that tells her what blondes are supposed to be. Blondes imply coolness because they are traditionally northern European, and northern Europeans are more repressed. There is a tendency to put this kind of woman on a pedestal."

Dr. Symonds believes that women who color their hair can have either a healthy or a neurotic motivation.

She characterizes healthy motivation as that caused by the woman's desire to enhance her looks and life.

She terms color change neurotic when blonding is done with great anxiety, as if color alone will make a radical difference in a woman's life.

UCLA psychiatrist Dr. Roderic Gorney takes quite another point of view. He dedicates a section of his book, *The Human Agenda* (the Guild of Tutors Press, Los Angeles, 1979 third edition), to what he calls "the quest for blondeness."

He ties in the adulation of blondes with, among other things, love of daylight and fear of nighttime darkness. He claims that the blonde image has come to connote both childhood innocence and sexual abandon in females.

"Despite occasional apparent exceptions, the blonde image is not mysterious, devious, or threatening. It depicts the heroine, not the heavy. For example, even in Harlow's gun moll roles, you knew that she was really a good girl underneath and that given half a chance she would have done right," he writes.

Dr. Sidney Kleinman, a psychoanalyst, sees these divergent views of blondes presenting problems for many women. "The blonde with two seemingly opposite images in conflict—the self-yearning for innocence and purity on one hand, and the external, sexual, forbidden-fruit image on the other— must reconcile them," he asserts.

"All women are struggling with this, but in the blonde it is more obvious. Women question how sensual, sexual and physical they can be and still maintain their self-worth. What the blonde must attempt is to integrate those two impulses so that she can continue as the repository of softer, more tender emotions and at the same time be open to her sexuality—seeing both as aspects of life-affirming behavior."

Dr. Kleinman believes that the blonde woman whose lightness represents purity even as she projects a forbidden-fruit image to men will be in the forefront of behavior patterns that will influence all women. "The way the blonde manages to integrate the two impulses can eventually provide the model whereby all women will reconcile their innocence and sensuality," he said.

But as women struggle to "reconcile their innocence and sensuality," men seem to have made up their minds.

In focus group interviews conducted in 1979 under the direction of David L. Schneider, Ph.D., men were asked for an immediate response to blondes versus brunettes. The men, ranging in age from their late 20's to their early 40's, included both white-collar and blue-collar workers. Their first reaction to the blonde woman was sexual.

Said one, "To me a blonde means good times and better sex."

Other responses were "easy to score," "sensual."

In still another test Dr. Schneider asked separate panels of men and women to give one-word descriptions of twelve different pictures of blonde women.

Eight out of the twelve pictures evoked the same response from both men and women.

Conditioned as we all are by movies, television and The Blonde Myth that begins in childhood, it is not surprising that both men and women found the same pictures "cute" or "cold" or "seductive."

In talking about blondes, neither men nor women differentiated between the light and pale blondes or the darker-toned blondes. Anything that didn't come across as brunette or redhead was "blonde."

But is blonde just a color?

Barbaralee Diamonstein, a blonde writer, lecturer and television personality in the arts world, doesn't think so. She believes that blonde is not a color but a state of mind.

"I think that others think about blondeness more than those who actually are blonde," said Ms. Diamonstein. "Other people remind us all the time that there is a myth, and I suppose after a while we think so, too." She paused and then added, "I don't think about being blonde, but I have been one, first by nature, and then by choice, all of my life."

"There is, of course, an anti-intellectual perception of blondeness," said this intellectual blonde. "There's the feeling that if one becomes blonde, it is a response to the hype. I don't feel that way. If being blonde makes you feel good—and colors your self-esteem, if only for weeks at a time—I think that's terrific.

"Being blonde is not low-brow or low-minded. It's also not an irrevocable decision."

Do Blondes Have More Fun?

Dr. Gorney believes that blonde women give the impression of joyousness partly because they are living up to expectations inculcated over a long period of time. "Because of that expectation, blondes tend to smile more, laugh more and act more vivacious. But inside they may not really be more joyous," he said.

Bette Midler has a less scientific answer. "Blondes do have more fun, but it's hell keeping up with the black roots."

Dr. Joyce Brothers says that being blonde made a difference in her life. "All the studies show that blondes really do have more fun. We don't necessarily get more men in terms of marriage but this is because there are more brunettes which weights the statistics. But a blonde does get more attention."

When women who haven't been blonde change their hair color, they often change the way they feel about themselves.

Susan Saint James, the actress whose natural brown hair was stripped and dyed blonde for a movie role, said in a "Good Morning America" interview, "I loved the way I looked when it was finished. Let me tell you, blonde's the way to go. I used to drive a pickup truck, but I couldn't as a blonde. I started driving a Seville because I loved the way it looked. But finally," she admitted, "I went back to being brown-haired because being blonde was too much trouble."

For some women it's worth the trouble.

Faith Brunson, a well-known Atlanta businesswoman, let her hair go gray. One day, at a friend's insistence, she colored it back to its original blonde shade.

"I couldn't believe the reactions of people," she said. "I got such a kick out of people telling me I looked the way I did twenty years ago. And each time I passed a mirror, I wondered who that blonde could be. Being blonde again made me feel happy."

Still there are blondes who insist that their hair color is not a part of their self-image. Charlotte Ford is one of them. "The only time I was really aware of being a blonde was when I visited Russia," she said. "I was fascinated to see every head turn when I walked by. It wasn't because of who I am. It was because most Russians are dark-haired. They couldn't believe that the long blonde hair on my head was real. They couldn't stop looking."

Another woman who found that people couldn't stop looking is a good-looking blonde advertising executive who moved from Ohio to New York. Said Joellen Gerstenmeier, "Being a New York blonde is different from being blonde anyplace else. I'm from Ohio, but no one there treated blondes quite the way they do in New York."

"Blondes Sell": Halston

Pick up any magazine, tune in any TV show, and somewhere a blonde will be urging you to buy. Blonde models are hired to sell lipstick, soap, perfume and clothes.

Cheryl Tiegs sells everything from cigarettes to automobiles to hair color. Farrah Fawcett sells shampoo. Margaux Hemingway was given a million dollars to launch a fragrance. Ditto for Candice Bergen with still another fragrance house. And what about Catherine Deneuve and the beautiful blonde personality she gave to Chanel No. 5? Lauren Hutton and Cheryl Ladd and Suzanne Somers—they're all blonde, and they all have advertising clients.

Why are so many blondes used in the media?

The award-winning designer Halston puts it succinctly, "Blondes sell."

Wilhelmina, the former model who now runs her own model agency with her husband, Bruce Cooper, says, "When you deal with people west of the Hudson, as we in our business do, you want that healthy, all-American look. That's what American women want to look like and a lot of blondes seem to have it." Wilhelmina stresses that none of her models looks phony.

"Models don't wear false eyelashes, false nails or hairpieces anymore, and they don't spend all their time in beauty salons." Wilhelmina's blonde models who color their hair want to look real. "That natural streaky look is in fashion now," Wilhelmina states authoritatively. The streaky look, also known as dimensional blonding, is that subtle interplay of light and darker blonde shades. Wilhelmina stays away from the very light, bright blondes. "That look doesn't sell in our business. In fact, if a girl has very light hair, I ask her to put dark streaks in it or it looks bleached even if it isn't."

And Wilhelmina has proved again and again that she has a good eye when it comes to finding all-American beauties. It was Wilhelmina who discovered top blonde model Patti Hanson.

Nina Blanchard, head of her own model agency in Los Angeles, notes, "About seventy-five percent of our calls are for blondes. It's never been any other way."

Fashion photographer Ara Gallant figures blondes have "a more approachable, open image."

Henry Wolf, the photographer/designer, whose work has appeared in *Harper's Bazaar* and *Vogue*, probes deeper for the reason so many blonde models are used. "It's all a part of the idealized latent images we have," he says. "The images are implanted early. We wait for the real thing to happen, and when it does it's like a camera where the images fuse, and *zap!* We spend all our lives programing what we consider beautiful, and the object all through life is to get close to the original *zap*.

"But beauty," says Henry Wolf wistfully, "is like love. The moment of attainment is the beginning of decline."

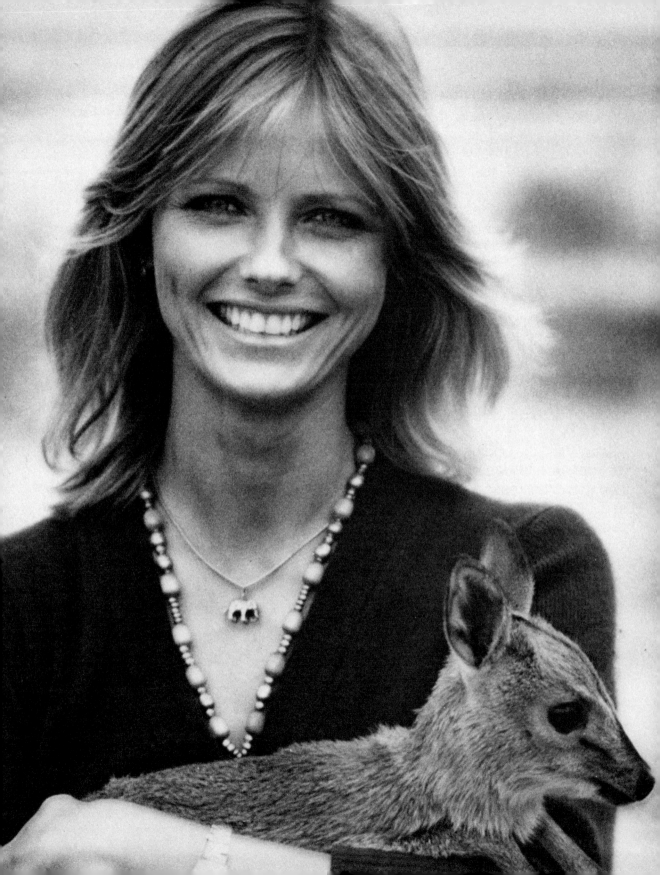

The Long Blonde Line

"Blondes are favorites
in every species.
Look at the animal kingdom.
Everyone thinks the lion
is the king of the jungle.
We look at the lion's mane
as a thing of beauty.
We don't talk the same way
about the rhino or the panther,
and they're both smarter
and more interesting animals
than the lion."

Cheryl Tiegs

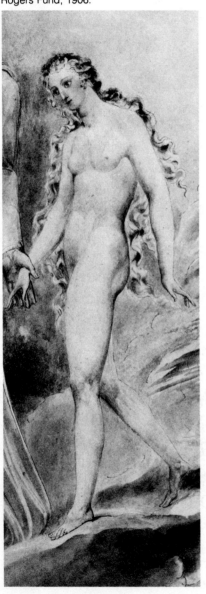

Detail of Eve from *She shall be called Woman*
by William Blake.
The Metropolitan Museum of Art,
Rogers Fund, 1906.

It All Started with Eve

According to the Talmud, the first two women in the world were blondes. Not only was Eve a blonde, but also Lilith, whom the Talmud calls Adam's first wife.

Wars have been fought over blondes, beginning with Helen of Troy whose beauty supposedly precipitated the Trojan War. And at 40, legend has it, Helen was still so beautiful that when she was ordered executed, the executioner was told to blindfold himself so he wouldn't be unduly dazzled by her looks.

Even Cleopatra, the famed Queen of the Nile, was a blonde. What about the black hair we always see on her? Ah, that was a wig that the lady, a strawberry blonde, always wore.

Other early beauties were Messalina, who ruled Rome when her husband, Claudius, was emperor; Simonetta Vespucci, the beloved of Giuliano de' Medici, brother of Lorenzo the Magnificent, who was described as being "especially beautiful and having winding ringlets on her golden head"; Lady Godiva, the eleventh-century Englishwoman who attempted to convince her husband that the townspeople's taxes were unjust by riding through Coventry wearing nothing but her long blonde hair; Queen Isabella, the monarch who arranged Columbus's voyage.

Lucrezia Borgia came along in the Middle Ages, and although she is reputed to have poisoned her enemies, she had an army of lovers. Her hair, described by a writer as "bright gold," was once cut and given to a lover, a poet named Bembo, and after 500 years that hair is still in the possession of his family.

Royalty paid homage to its blondes all through history. For instance, there were Anne of Austria, wife of Louis XIII, and the three blonde mistresses of Louis XIV, the Sun King: Louise de la Vallière, who later became a Carmelite nun; the Duchesse de Fontanges, who introduced the fashion of a ribbon around the head; and the Marquise de Maintenon, who eventually became the king's wife.

The blonde Madame de Pompadour was Louis XV's mistress for twenty years, and battled Church and State to rule France. Legend has it that she was also a woman of wit and humor. As the priest who was administering the last rites prepared to take his leave, Madame de Pompadour managed to say with a small smile, "What a hurry you are in, Monsieur. Wait a while, and we will go together."

The next mistress of Louis XV was also a blonde, the famed Madame du Barry. And Louis XVI's queen was the even more famous blonde, Marie Antoinette, who never did say those famous words, "Let them eat cake."

Mademoiselle Fel, the famous blonde opera singer of the 1700's, was both friend and confidante to La Tour, the painter; Kitty Fisher, one of the most celebrated and intelligent courtesans in English history, was a blonde—of course. So was La Belle O'Morphi, daughter of an Irish shoemaker who at thirteen was seduced by Casanova and later was immortalized in the paintings of Boucher.

Lady Caroline Lamb, with her curly golden hair, caught the eye of Lord Byron, and other ladies with literary connections include Letitia Elizabeth Landon, who under the pen name of "L.E.L." became one of England's most successful poets.

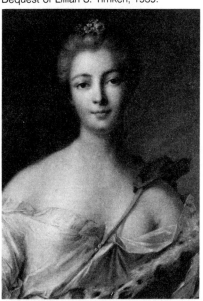

Detail from *Madame de Pompadour as Diana* by Jean Marc Nattier.
The Metropolitan Museum of Art,
Bequest of Lillian S. Timken, 1959.

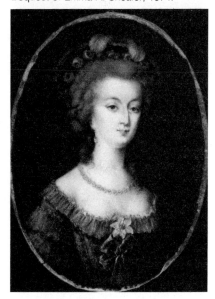

Detail from *Marie Antoinette* by imitator of Louise Elisabeth Vigee-Le Brun.
The Metropolitan Museum of Art,
Bequest of Emma A. Sheafer, 1974.

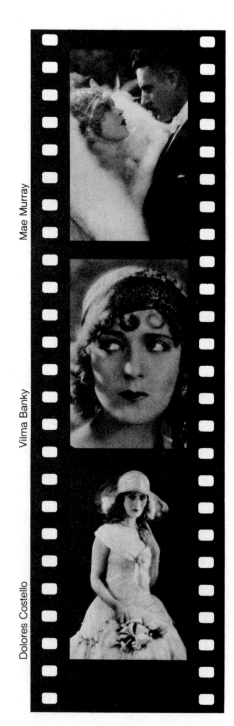

Mae Murray

Vilma Banky

Dolores Costello

The Movie Blondes

Today's blonde heroines come not from the world of art or literature, but from the television tube or the movie house.

They had their genesis in early Hollywood and the success of Mary Pickford who established herself as "the sweet young thing."

Mary Pickford was so popular that when D. W. Griffith, the famous Biograph movie director, took the film's first close-up using Pickford as the subject, the front office complained. "The audiences pay more to see Mary's films. They should be privileged to see *all* of her."

After Mary Pickford came a long line of beautiful blondes.

There were Bessie Barriscale, a silent-screen star, who in those days played both sweet maidens *and* sultry vamps; Texas Guinan, who, besides her New York night club activities, also played in serials; Mae Murray, who was best known for her bee-stung lips; Vilma Banky, whose lavish wedding in the 1920's to fellow screen star Rod La Rocque was staged by Samuel Goldwyn; Lilyan Tashman, who for years until her tragic death at the height of her career held the title of "the best-dressed movie star in the film capital"; Dolores Costello, the woman John Barrymore demanded as a co-star (he got her both as a co-star and as a wife); Marion Davies, who began as a dancer in the 1918 Ziegfeld Follies, became the first Hollywood star to have a portable dressing room and is best remembered for her alliance with William Randolph Hearst.

Other major blondes in early film days were Lillian Gish, Greta Garbo, Ann Harding and Constance Bennett. Constance's sister, Joan, was the only Hollywood blonde who became a star as a brunette. That change of color prompted Cole Porter to write, Let's talk of Lamarr—that Hedy so fair—why does she let Joan Bennett—wear all her old hair?''

The Platinum Blonde, Jean Harlow, was Hollywood's first real sex-symbol blonde. But despite her sexy, happy on-screen performance, she was most sedate off-screen. She got her big chance in "Hell's Angels," when producer Howard Hughes, who had just finished making a silent version of the film, had to do it all over again because his leading lady, a Continental star, had a foreign accent.

Jean Harlow was an instant star, and according to one poll she rose from total obscurity to "the eighteenth best-known person in the world" within a year. Her hits included "Red Dust," "Riff-Raff," "Bombshell," "Dinner at Eight" and "Platinum Blonde." At the height of her popularity Hollywood introduced its own Production Code, and the title of a Harlow film was changed from "Born to Be Kissed" to "The Girl from Missouri."Hollywood was always experimenting with Harlow, and at one point (for "Riff-Raff") she darkened her hair, and the studio did a big publicity campaign on "Harlow Going Brownette." She was back to platinum for her next picture.

She died at the age of 26, and years later a biography by Irving Shulman called *Harlow* (Bernard Geis Associates, Inc., 1964) analyzed her effect on America. In the book Shulman said, "Jean Harlow was the woman who typified the distinctive, unique type of American beauty, which has since been imitated throughout the world. Succeeding decades have modified that beauty, but basically it is gay, carefree, healthy and athletic, wholesomely sexual without being furtive or dirty. And always it is blonde."

After Harlow came Thelma Todd, who, although she

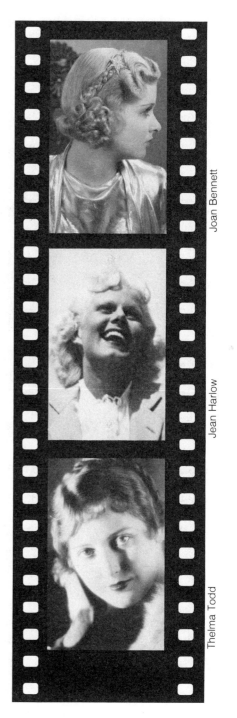

Joan Bennett

Jean Harlow

Thelma Todd

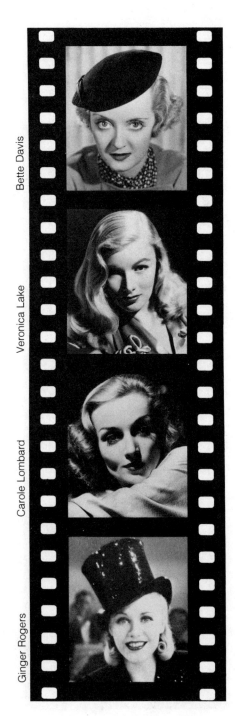

Bette Davis

Veronica Lake

Carole Lombard

Ginger Rogers

played flashy blonde roles, was a proper New England girl; Carole Landis, whose early film "Four Jills and a Jeep" still shows up on late-night TV; Joan Blondell, an early portrayer of the not-so-dumb blonde gold digger; Miriam Hopkins, the blonde who was as well known for her feud with Bette Davis as for her acting talent. Bette Davis was very blonde in most of her major movies from "Jezebel" to "Baby Jane," and she was practically white-blonde when she uttered that great line, "Ah'd love to kiss you, but Ah just washed my hair." Then we can't forget Sonja Henie, the ice skater, who glided head-to-toe right into everyone's heart; Simóne Simon, the French import, who taught America a thing or two about European blondes (they're just as glamorous); Veronica Lake, the actress who wore her hair over one eye, introducing the most imitated hair style in the history of the country. That hair style actually caused a crisis in World War II production, because women who worked in defense factories were so busy copying it they endangered their lives: their hair was always getting caught in the machinery.

Then there were Grace Moore, the only opera star who successfully made the transition from the Met to films; Carole Lombard, the most gifted comedienne of her time; Mae West, the boisterous blonde with the terrific sense of humor, whose famous line, "Come up and see me sometime" has never been forgotten; Ginger Rogers, who went from dancing to serious acting and wound up with an Oscar (for "Kitty Foyle" in 1940).

Betty Grable, the hottest pin-up in World War II, found that happy and blonde were not necessarily synonymous. She was once described as America's ideal girl. (In those days the terms "ideal" and "girl" had no sexist overtones. "Ideal" referred to her measurements which were 34-23-35. And as for "girl," she inspired the song "I Want a Girl Just Like the Girl Who Married Harry James," the bandleader who was then her husband.)

Marlene Dietrich, once described as "a Wall Street mind in a Broadway chassis," was an early blonde beauty and made her mark in Josef von Sternberg's "Blue Angel." Lana Turner, who really was discovered drinking a Coke in Schwab's drugstore, became the Sweater Girl and a blonde ideal for millions of men and women. Marie Wilson was a famous "dumb blonde" type who for years starred in Ken Murray's "Blackouts" revue and then became TV's "My Friend Irma." Betty Hutton symbolized the happy-go-lucky personality blonde, and—like many other stars—her real life was a painful contrast to the bubbly personality she portrayed on screen.

Gold diggers (the role was generally a hard-boiled glamour girl) were popular in the twenties and thirties, and almost always they were blonde. In addition to Harlow, Mae West and the late Joan Blondell, there were gold diggers like Wendy Barrie, Lilyan Tashman and Glenda Farrell. (Blondell once did a movie, "Blondie Johnson," and Dietrich was the world's "Blonde Venus.") Barbara Stanwyck frequently played the toughie with a heart of gold, but for the roles in which she was really vicious with no heart at all ("Double Indemnity" and "Baby Face") she went blonde. And, of course, she turned blonde to star in "Stella Dallas," the greatest tearjerker of them all.

A brunette song-and-dance girl, Dorothy McNulty, played minor roles until she went blonde, changed both her personality and her name (Penny Singleton), and today is best-known as "Blondie."

Although Groucho Marx's heart really belonged to Margaret Dumont, he was always following his cigar in the direction of blondes like Thelma Todd and Esther

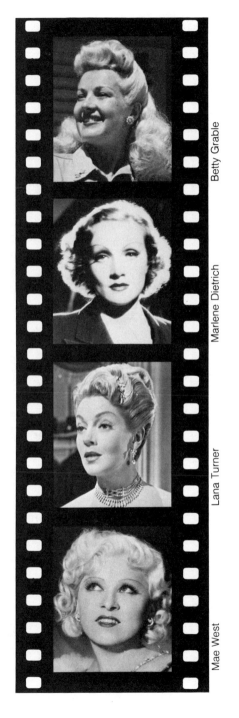

Betty Grable

Marlene Dietrich

Lana Turner

Mae West

23

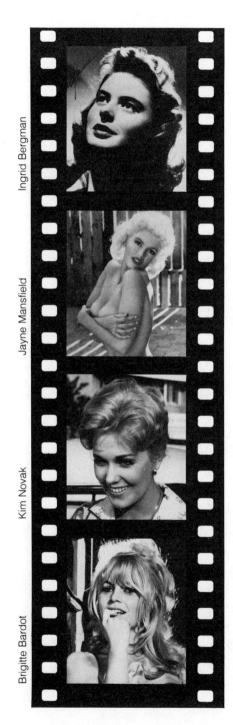

Ingrid Bergman

Jayne Mansfield

Kim Novak

Brigitte Bardot

Muir, while Harpo constantly chased the cute Toby Wing type of blonde.

The "Topper" series was a smash in films when blonde Constance Bennett played the glamorous ghost. And it worked on television when blonde Anne Jeffreys played the role. But the TV "Topper" special was a disaster—and it was the only time a brunette was given the lead.

Ann Sothern played in 25 different "Maisie" movies, and in each she was a blonde who outsmarted everyone. Ingrid Bergman was the sophisticated blonde who made worldwide headlines when she cut her thick blonde hair after the film "Intermezzo" for a role that made her even more famous, Maria, in "For Whom the Bell Tolls."

But the most elegant blonde of all was Grace Kelly, born to play the part of Tracy Lord in "Philadelphia Story," but who won an Academy Award in 1954 for her role opposite Bing Crosby in "Country Girl."

Following the regal looks of Grace Kelly came some well-known sex kittens: Jayne Mansfield, who loved everything pink and even had a pink swimming pool; and Janet Leigh, who later became famous as the woman in the shower in the film "Psycho"; Kim Novak, who once tinted her blonde hair purple; and Anita Ekberg, a tall and sexy Swedish blonde. Eva Marie Saint began with the usual Hollywood pin-up ballyhoo of her generation and went on to become better known for her acting than her cheesecake photos. And who can forget Brigitte Bardot with her bee-stung lips, tousled hair and French bikini?

Bob Hope did a lot to extend the blonde image when in the late 30's and 40's he told countless blonde jokes—all with the beautiful Madeline Carroll, the actress, as the foil. One of Hope's big movies at the time was "My Favorite Blonde" with Madeline Carroll.

Judy Holliday was the first of the wide-eyed blondes with a mind like a computer. Goldie Hawn is the latest.

The blondes who made families famous were the Gabors. Mama Jolie and her daughters, Zsa Zsa and Eva, have been as well known for their headline marriages as their hairline colors.

But no other blonde ever had the impact wielded by Marilyn Monroe. She began as a pin-up girl but became a fine comedienne, and, as every reader of magazines must know, Marilyn married two of the most famous (and different) men of her time, Joe DiMaggio and Arthur Miller. In death, as in life, she exerts an almost mystical power over people.

Marilyn Monroe, like all blondes who soar to superstar status, has that dichotomy Dr. Gorney referred to as both "innocence and sexual abandon."

And so goes that duality with blondes. No one ever talks about a fickle brunette, a dumb brunette—yet those descriptions are used with blonde. If the lady is blonde, we seem to know a lot of blonde putdowns. Yet when she's regarded positively, her hair color is never mentioned.

The next chart illustrates:

Trait	Positive	Negative
A fondness for change.	Flexibility	Fickle blonde
An inclination to be domineering.	Executive talent	Bossy blonde
A desire to be noticed.	Glamour	Flashy blonde
A tendency to be a good mixer.	Friendliness	Dumb blonde
A compulsion to have many irons in the fire.	Energy	Dizzy blonde
A value for money.	Business sense	Gold-digging blonde

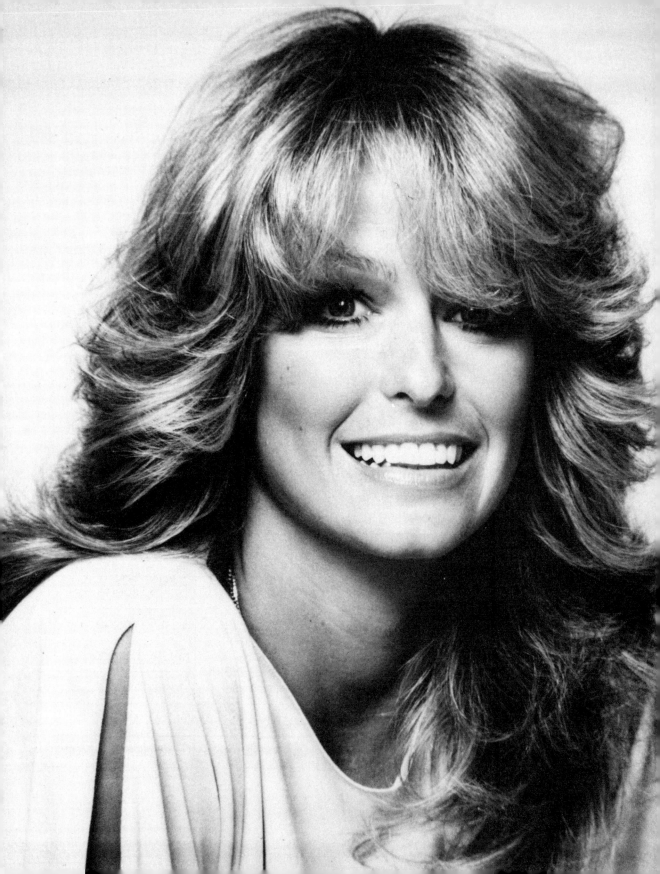

The Blonde Advantage

"In theatre, the adage of
the knowing actor has always been,
'Never step on stage with a dog or a kid.'
The shrewd actors expand the taboo list
to include blonde actresses."

Lee Guber

Farrah Fawcett: the blonde who symbolized the glamour of the '70's

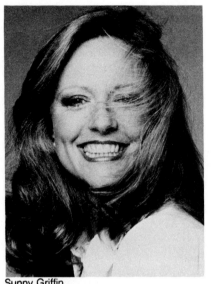
Sunny Griffin

Maybe theatrical producer Lee Guber's observation accounts for the reason that most of the legendary stage stars are brunette. Everyone's willing to share the stage with them. Duse, Katharine Cornell, Lynn Fontanne, and Ethel Merman were all known for their strong, dark looks. On the other hand, natural brunettes like Ethel Barrymore, Helen Hayes, Tallulah Bankhead, Mary Martin and Ina Claire all lightened their hair at some time during their careers. Jeanne Eagels, more famous for her stormy and tragic private life than for most of her stage roles (although she was Sadie Thompson in "Rain") was blonde and grew blonder. So did some of the best of the more recent stage actresses, women like Geraldine Page, Kim Stanley and Meryl Streep.

Roles are played differently when the heroine is blonde, and that's true off stage, too. Lee Guber says that blondes, both off-stage and on-stage, play every role like a star. He adds, "If a woman doesn't want to go blonde, she should at least think blonde so her audience won't be able to take its eyes off her."

Cathi Hunt of Clairol agrees that there is indeed a blonde mentality. "The woman who thinks blonde always believes she's prettier and more attractive."

Women who are blonde know that blonding is a high.

Sunny Griffin of Avon admits, "Whenever I get down in the dumps, I go to Robert Renn, my colorist, and say, 'Make me blonder.'"

More than a woman's psyche can hinge on hair color. François, the New York hair stylist, tells of a woman whose roots are colored every two weeks so that her husband, who married her as a blonde, will never know about her dark past.

Both men and women are caught up in The Blonde Myth.

Michael Stinchcomb, the colorist at Yves Claude Hair in New York, thinks deep down all women want to be blonde. "When a woman is blonde," he theorizes, "she feels more attractive. She has more of a feeling of glamour."

Chances of a blonde's changing to brunette are slim. Colorists everywhere agree that changing a blonde back to brunette is a traumatic experience for the client. Virginia Graham, head colorist at Vidal Sassoon, Beverly Hills, says that when it's necessary to stop blonding for a customer, "I know I'm going to be in trouble, and she's not going to like me because she's going to hate losing her blondeness, and her husband is going to hate it, too."

Why do men prefer blondes?

Graham has her own reasons: "I think blonde women tend to act flightier, which makes men feel more masculine."

Jill Hee, consumer relations manager at Clairol, notes, "If a woman has a marriage problem, her first response—after 'Kill the other woman'—is 'I'll be a blonde.' Women feel being blonde gives them a competitive advantage."

Susan Silver agrees. She came to California to write a movie script. "My hair was somewhere between dark blonde and brown, so I added a few streaks. The first time I went to a restaurant the owner came over to tell me how fantastic I looked. I *felt* fantastic. He didn't know what it was. But I did. I know that when you're blonde in California you feel a lot better about yourself."

Rose Reti, the famous New York colorist, agrees. But she thinks blonde makes women feel better regardless of the city. Rose Reti, a soft-spoken blonde ("I was always blonde. Even as a baby, I was blonde"), was born in Hungary, spent a lifetime in the beauty business and today runs her own salon on New York's East Side. Her clients include Dina Merrill, the Gabors, Barbara de Portago, Joyce Susskind, Jill Haworth and *the* cover girl of the 1950's, Jean Patchett.

"Women became blonde back in the days when Florenz Ziegfeld made the blonde woman the desirable one," she recalled. "In the 1930's women were blonde because they followed fashion, and fashion was blonde. In the 1940's life was hard because we had a war so we needed something to cheer people up. What cheers people more than a blonde woman?"

In 1954 Rose Reti made Zsa Zsa Gabor blonde for her role in "Moulin Rouge," and later she turned sister Eva blonde for "Happy Time," the play in which she co-starred with Paul Lukas on Broadway.

But what's the first step? How do women indicate they want blonding when they enter a salon?

"It's very simple," Rose Reti says with a small shrug. "They don't even have to ask for blonding. A woman comes in. She is low in spirit and wants to look glamorous. I know she means blonde. So I say, 'What about a few highlights?' And so it begins.

"Blonding gives a woman a lift. It makes her feel good. When I go out at night to a restaurant with my husband, I don't go as a professional in the beauty business. I go just like any other wife, and I sit and watch the people. That's what I like best, just watching the people. Women come into the restaurant, and men's eyes follow them. Of course they don't follow all women, but the ones who make the men sit up straight and look at them first are the blondes.

"Clothes today are made for blondes. The whole light look is a blonde look. Chiffon and crepe de chine, those are for blondes.

"Not everyone should be blonde," Miss Rose is quick to say. "When I made Joan Crawford blonde, for a movie role, it washed her out."

Miss Rose will not change every woman who asks.

She shakes her head sadly. "Some women don't understand. When a woman comes into the salon and asks for me, I have her seated so I can study her without her knowing. Then I go out to meet her. I watch her stand up. If she walks heavy, she cannot be a blonde. She doesn't have to be thin to be blonde, but she can't walk heavy. To that woman I say, 'A few light brown streaks for you.'

"Also a woman must have a life style to support her blonde look. She has to have the budget and be able to come to the salon.

"Sometimes I watch women after they have color. They smile. They are happy. They are young."

But even though recaptured youth is the rainbow women chase, not all men want their wives to look young. Most do, but Miss Rose has one client married to a man fifteen years her senior. He wants her to have gray hair so she won't look too young to be his wife.

Miss Rose will not make a dark brunette blonde. As a dark brunette goes gray, Miss Rose gives her light brown highlights. "All women need a little something," she says with a small nod of her head.

"After a certain age a woman seeks attention. Perhaps she has been neglected by her husband or children. Maybe she isn't appreciated in her job. She wants someone to take time with her. We do that."

Generally Miss Rose believes that the older a woman is, the better she looks as a blonde because blonde is not so far from gray.

The youngest person she has ever made blonde was a 14-year-old appearing in a Broadway show. The oldest? An 89-year-old woman whose name she will never reveal. "An 89-year-old woman is entitled to her secrets," Miss Rose says gently.

Blonde According to Blanchard

Leslie Blanchard is a famous hair colorist who's interested in adding color to lives as well as hair. He says "I will never color a woman's hair until I talk to her. I must know something of her life. I want to know her reason for color. Of course, I never get the real reason the first time I ask, but after a few minutes I'll know why the woman wants it."

Other Blanchard philosophies:

"The biggest mistake women make is to ask, 'What will hair color do for me?'

"A woman can't expect her hair to move, talk and walk for her. The excitement comes from within. You can't lie back and let your hair do all the work.

"I'm not sure I know all the reasons women become blonde, but gray is the last reason.

"The best reason for color is when a woman says to herself that she isn't quite as good as she can be and wants color to heighten her feelings about herself.

"A lot of women who aren't really blonde have a blonde look.

"I color Barbara Walters's hair. She's an example of a woman whose hair is really brown but who now has a blonde look. For Barbara it's an individual, sophisticated look and right for her life.

"Some people don't know what blonde really means in terms of color.

"Blonde doesn't mean no color. Quite the opposite. Blonde means lightness, softness, delicacy, airiness.

"Women should be different kinds of blondes or have different colors at different times in their lives.

"At 18 a woman can do anything; it's always right.

"From 18 to 25 she can experiment.

"At 25 it's time to cool it, find an area that will work best.

"From 25 to 35 she can have an exciting, high-key look and make the most of every part of herself.

"After 35 it's time to enjoy what you have and modify the look that's most successful for you. At this time a woman should not be seeking out but adding to—it's the plus time of life.

"After 50 the woman should be behind the spotlight, not under it, except for those moments when she really wants the spotlight. After 50 it's time to enjoy your success and not be frantic and harassed in search of yourself.

"Blonde hair can really make you something.

"Without blonde, a woman can be just another pretty face, and pretty faces are a dime a dozen. Blondeness seems to give a woman an inside camera so she becomes not what you see but what she sees and expresses of herself.

"Thank heaven we've taken women off pedestals.

"We did that in the 1960's and 1970's. We had to show that women were not just glossy, but now that women have proved they're gutsy, too, they can go back to being pretty in the 1980's."

What Kind of Blonde Are You?

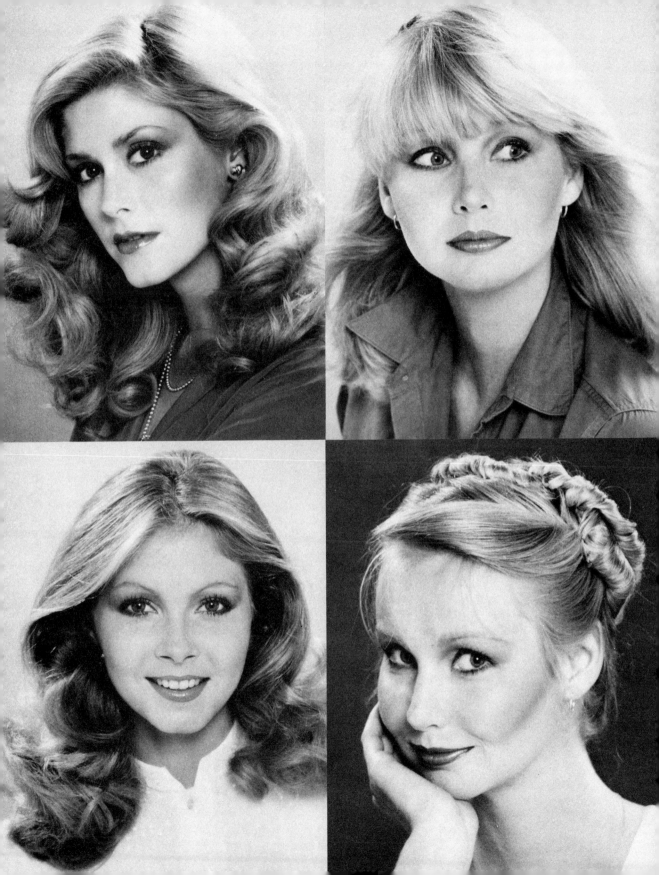

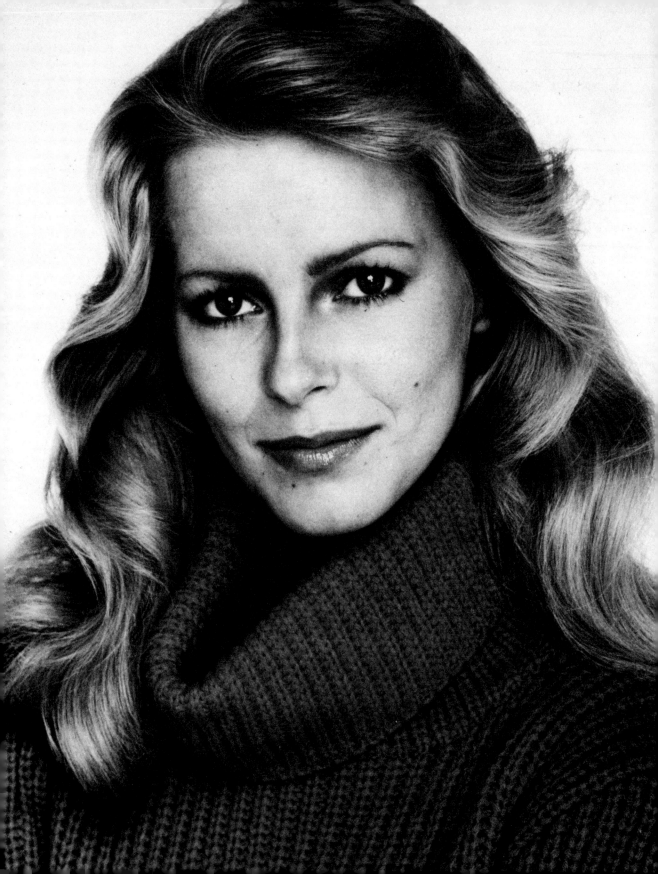

The Best Blonde Looks

*"When you're hot, you're hot.
And 27-year-old Cheryl Ladd
is about as hot these days
as a multimedia star can get.
She's also a living reminder that
blonde hair, blue eyes, and white teeth
are still the American media's
—specifically television's—
most marketable commodities."*

Peter Funt,
Cue *magazine, May 11, 1979*

Cheryl Ladd: another blonde angel

When we talk about redheads most of us focus on a single image: The hair is red, and the personality fiery. Brunette means dark hair and a sultry woman.

But blonde means many things.

It means young and not so young.

It means different parts of the country.

It means different temperaments, different personalities.

That's why a blonde book must explore different kinds of blonde.

I think there are five different blonde types. There's the woman who looks as if she's born to be blonde, has the cool, Nordic, ice-princess look. I call her the Scandinavian Blonde.

The young, fresh, outdoorsy, streaky blonde is the purest California Blonde.

When a woman is over 21, blonde and a chic urban career woman, she is the New York Blonde.

The Palm Beach Blonde is the sophisticated woman of means, who wears her blondeness like her diamonds.

And the Newport Blonde epitomizes the best of the relaxed, secure exurban blonde.

The Scandinavian Blonde

Ingrid Bergman was an early example of this kind of beauty; Liv Ullmann is a present-day Scandinavian blonde.

She is the woman who looks as if she grew and bloomed farm-fresh in the North Country. It's this look that the writer Lafcadio Hearn described as "a reflection of celestial loveliness . . . because it bears . . . the suggestion of force, will, strength and loyalty—the glory of the North—cold, fresh, strong and immortal."

The Scandinavian Blonde is born to the look. Her

hair is very very blonde. In childhood it's almost white. Then in her teens it deepens to a golden blonde and darkens further as she gets older. She's often blue-eyed and white-skinned. Although she may be warm-hearted, her cool, crisp look sets her apart and often makes people think she's aloof and uninterested in others.

This is frequently the blonde style Americans prefer when they talk about true blondes.

Eileen Ford agrees. The head of the famous Ford Models, Inc. says, "I don't know why, but I guess Americans like to think they look Scandinavian. When a client calls up and says, 'Give me a classic all-American girl,' I know what he means is someone like the Danish models we have."

The California Blonde

There's a rumor, fostered no doubt by the California Chamber of Commerce, that no woman who's short, brunette and fat is allowed to enter California. Brunettes evidently are put into a sealed room at the Los Angeles airport and then shipped back to their city of origin.

How else can you explain why all the women you see in California are blondes, and long, lithe ones at that, who always swing their hair?

California seems invented for the woman who surfs, runs on the beach and looks her best in short shorts.

Of course, the California Blonde can live anywhere in the world, but no matter where she lives, her look is athletic, fit.

She generally wears her hair shoulder length, and it always looks clean and shiny. It's not a pale blonde look that she has but rather the streaked look of a blonde who's played a lot of tennis—and played it well.

The Hemingway sisters are the California Blonde type: outdoor women, fresh and real.

Farrah Fawcett has the California look. She wears her hair like a blonde mane, then downplays the effects of her hair by wearing blue jeans, the true California touch.

And no matter where she travels, the California Blonde feels best in California.

The New York Blonde

The New York Blonde moves with assurance. She has made some difficult decisions and seems to be in command of her life. Her hair is very well cut and usually streaked; she is definitely not a one-shade blonde. Her clothes look as if she took both time and taste to assemble them. Her skin is clear, her eyes sparkle and she walks briskly in time to her own drummer.

Chances are she intensifies her blonde look with the aid of a very good colorist. As time goes by, her look becomes more and more blonde. Dr. Theodore Isaac Rubin believes that blonding for this woman is a signal, a symbolic gesture that she is doing something that will bring a big change in her life. Says Dr. Rubin, "Obviously the thing that can be changed easiest is the hair. In addition, a woman can have plastic surgery. She can even lose weight, but that takes too much time. For a small amount of time and money she can be blonde." Further he asserts that the woman who changes to blondeness believes she will have greater freedom to act out her femininity.

Often this woman is faced with a life crisis involving a loss, such as the end of a marriage through either death or divorce, the death of a parent, the loss of a job, or a move to a new city with the loss of old ties. She turns to blondeness as a signal to the outside world that she has decided to take things into her own hands for a second chance.

The Palm Beach Blonde

This is the woman who has come to terms with her look. She knows what to wear and how to wear it, and regardless of how the fashions may change, she stays in style.

She's tall, slim and may be over forty—but she doesn't look it.

She swims, but doesn't sun. She exercises, but doesn't play.

Her hair is cut close, and she visits a salon regularly. In addition to a haircut, she has her hair colored and gets regular facials and massages. She has probably had cosmetic surgery, for this is the blonde who is a disciplined beauty and is willing to pay the price to achieve her best look.

She is meticulous about herself, her home and her possessions. She has a passion for flowers, grows them in her own hothouse and is given to raising prize-winning orchids which decorate her home—but never her.

She is careful to answer all invitations promptly and has a wardrobe of monogrammed stationery: one with the name of her house (e.g., Happyland, The Palms), one with her name and his, one with her first name only and one with her formal married name.

You can spot a Palm Beach Blonde every time she opens her handbag because tucked in the corner is a real linen handkerchief edged in lace. A Palm Beach Blonde wouldn't be caught using tissues.

Of course, she doesn't have to live in Palm Beach to be a Palm Beach Blonde. She can be found any day not only on Worth Avenue but on the Champs Elysées,

Madison Avenue, Bond Street or Rodeo Drive, checking the shops, the galleries and the restaurants for the best of the newest.

The Newport Blonde

She's the woman who wears her blondeness as casually as her clothes. She's independent, bright, quick to laugh and has ready good manners. Her husband's successful and attractive; their tow-headed children are a delight. She's family oriented, loves sailing with all the family.

Nobody famous cuts her hair. She washes it herself and dries it in the air. And when the blondeness darkens or grays—well, so it's dark or gray.

She orders her favorite clothes from her favorite catalog: L. L. Bean. She and her husband have matching boots for duck hunting, matching sweaters for sailing.

She collects old ship accessories, has a freezer full of Girl Scout cookies and all the neighborhood children think she's the best mother around.

She belongs to her college alumnae association, may even be the class secretary. She's genuinely thoughtful and a sincere letter writer. In fact, for every occasion she sends notes that are easily recognizable because she hand writes them and is a master of calligraphy.

When she was a little girl she began riding in horse shows and can ride both English and Western saddle.

Her style is natural elegance.

Or, as Philip Barry wrote in *The Philadelphia Story,* she's yar.

Grace Kelly: the Newport Blonde in *High Society*
Photo: Culver Pictures

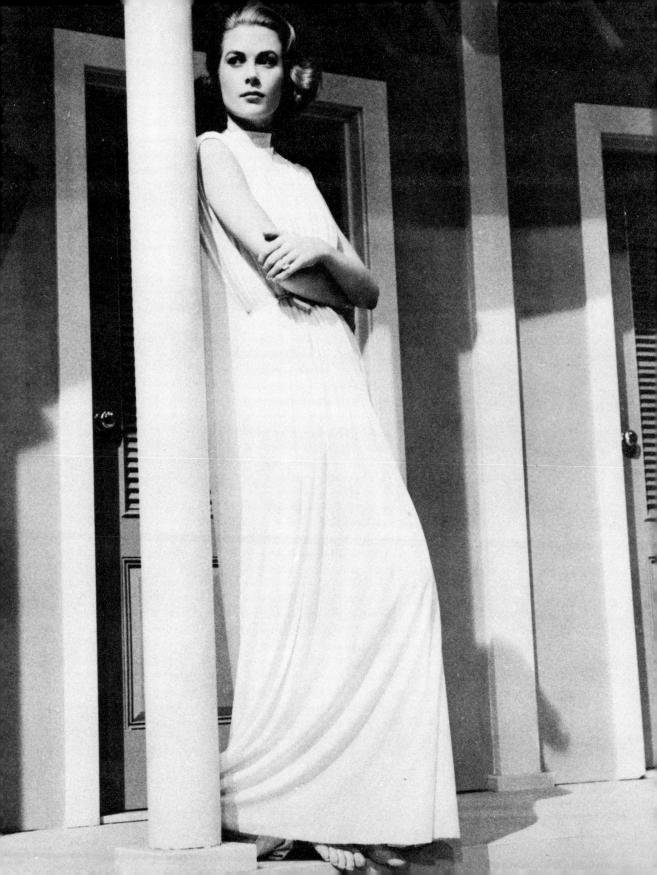

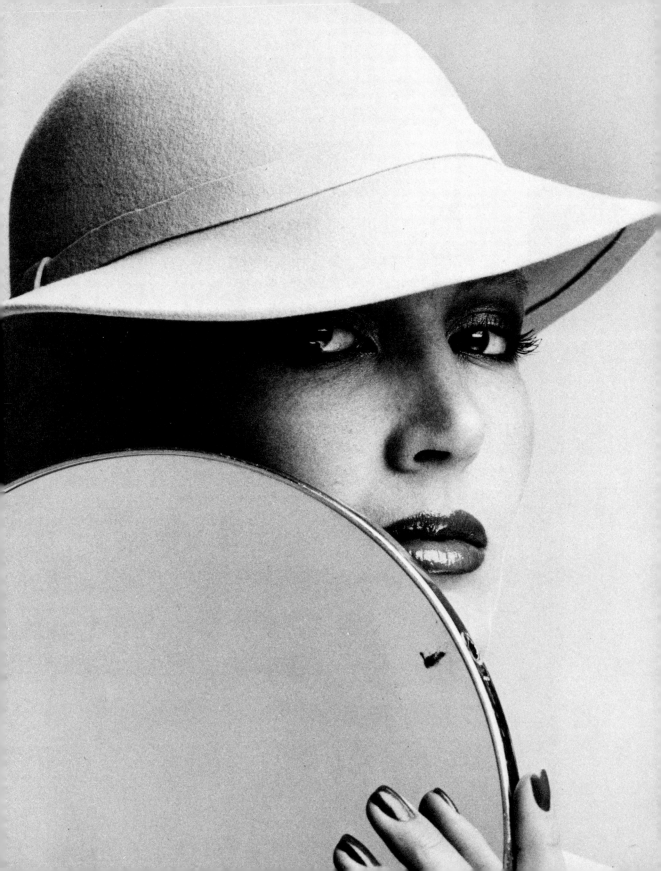

The Blonde Quiz

All right, so you've decided.
You're going to be pretty.
You're going blonde.
But what kind of blonde?

Blonde today is not a single statement, not a single look.

Blonde, like woman herself, is the result of options.

The key in blonding has always been to make the hair color work with the woman's overall skin tones, facial shape and general appearance. Much has been made of the relationship of color, cut and style to the face. Now there's another dimension to consider: life style.

No woman should color her hair either at home or in a salon without first knowing just how far she can go with color and remain psychologically comfortable with her new look.

There are three different types of *blonde personalities,* and before you color it's important to identify your own personality type in order to be able to choose the kind of blonding that will make you live happily ever after.

The test that follows will help you determine which type you are. Based on the results, there's a blonde way of life for you that matches your life style and your own opinions of yourself.

1. *You need something new in your wardrobe. You decide the next dress (or suit) you will buy will be*
   A. Bright colored: red, yellow, purple, orange
   B. Earth tones: beige, white, brown, black
   C. A replacement for something you now own

2. *An attractive man you've never met shows up at a friend's party. Would you*
   A. Go up to him and introduce yourself
   B. Ask the host (or hostess) to introduce you
   C. Wait for him to come over to meet you

3. *You hear via the grapevine that a job you want will be open in your company. Would you*
   A. Call the president's office and ask for the job

B. Ask your supervisor if you might apply

C. Hope someone will notice you and consider you

4. *The magazines you enjoy most are*
   A. *Glamour, Vogue, Mademoiselle, Cosmopolitan*
   B. *House Beautiful, Redbook, Good Housekeeping*
   C. *Time, Newsweek, Fortune, Forbes*

5. *The color of the most important room in your house is*
   A. Bright, lively, patterned
   B. Soft, subdued
   C. Not yet the color you want it to be

6. *The most important room in your house is*
   A. The bedroom
   B. The living room
   C. The kitchen

7. *How many lipsticks do you have?*
   A. Too many to count
   B. Three or four
   C. One or two

8. *Your eye makeup includes*
   A. Shadow, liner and mascara which you wear day and night
   B. Shadow day and evening; mascara only for big "dressy" nights
   C. Shadow at night only

9. *Your weight is*
   A. Within five pounds of where you want it
   B. Within ten pounds of where you want it
   C. More than ten pounds from perfect

10. *If you could have any car in the world, you'd choose*
    A. A Rolls-Royce Silver Cloud
    B. A Mercedes
    C. A BMW

11. *Your marital status is*
    A. Divorced or widowed
    B. Single
    C. Married
12. *Your favorite alcoholic drink is*
    A. White wine on the rocks
    B. Scotch or bourbon
    C. Martini
13. *Your favorite dance is*
    A. Disco
    B. The kind you did in high school
    C. Cheek-to-cheek
14. *You're having a dinner party. Would you include*
    A. Some new acquaintances who seem "interesting"
    B. Your spouse's (or your own) boss
    C. People who work in your (or your husband's) office
15. *It's vacation time. Would you*
    A. Take a trip alone to a foreign country
    B. Go on a cruise
    C. Go to a resort with a friend
16. *You're in New York for one evening. Would you*
    A. Go to Studio 54
    B. Go to the theater
    C. Go to a restaurant
17. *The waiter just brought the menu. He suggests the special of the day. You never heard of it. Would you*
    A. Go ahead and order it
    B. Ask the waiter to bring you an appetizer size so you can sample it
    C. Urge someone else at the table to try it
18. *You look in the mirror and see wrinkles around your eyes. Would you*
    A. Run to the phone and call a plastic surgeon
    B. Get new makeup

C. Shrug your shoulders and realize you're getting older
19. *You are buying new jeans. Would you choose*
    A. French or Italian jeans
    B. Calvin Klein, Gloria Vanderbilt or other de-
       signer jeans
    C. Bargain-basement jeans for $9.95
20. *Your best friend is*
    A. The most interesting person you know
    B. Someone you grew up with
    C. Your mother

   To find your type, give yourself three points for every
"A" answer, two for each "B" and one for each "C."
Add the total:

55-60/Type A Blondes are generally more adventurous, more willing to take a chance with life. This is
the woman who isn't afraid to be noticed, who goes out
of her way to meet opportunity. Dr. Ernst L. Wynder,
president of the American Health Foundation, profiles
this woman as one with an outgoing personality, sexually adventurous, more likely to read *Vogue* than *The
Atlantic,* inclined to be thin, probably a smoker, a social drinker (as opposed to abstainer).

40-55/Type B Blondes are women who want a different life but are concerned about the opinions of those
they love. They will take a chance but never at the risk
of losing self-esteem or the respect of those who matter to them. This is the woman who understands that
blondeness may represent the *beginning* of a new
identification but can never be the identification itself.

Under 40/Type C Blondes are women who want to
make a change—so long as it's not a radical change.
They are the women who are afraid of being regarded
as sex objects and are concerned with not only the
opinion of those they cherish but all opinion. This
woman avoids the limelight but is secretly romantic.

How To Achieve The Look You Want

Meryl Streep: blonde beauty was redefined for her look of the '80"

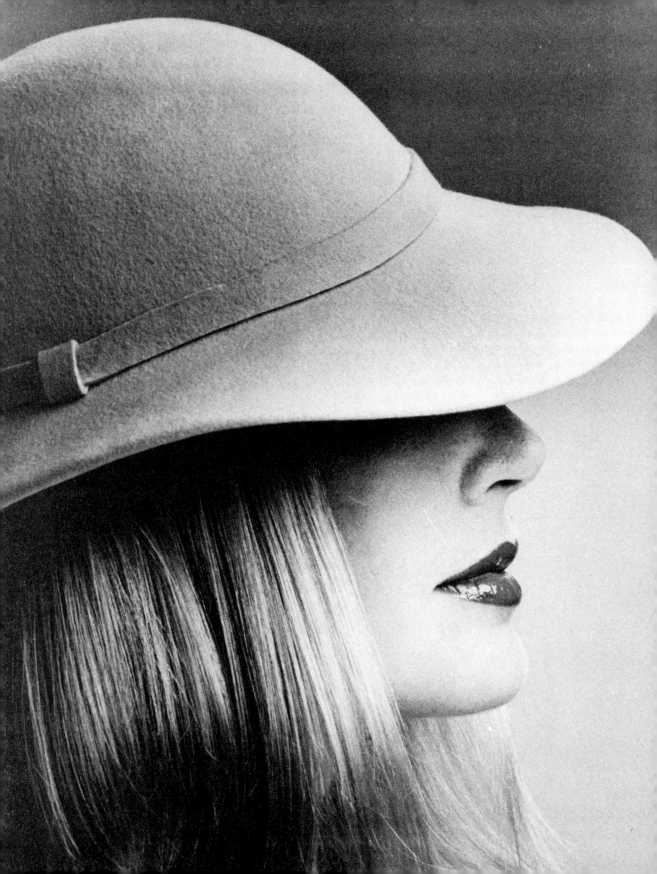

What To Know Before You Color

Q: How can you tell if a woman
should color her hair?

A: If she wears makeup,
she should color her hair.

Dominic Durastanti

It's only in the last 35 years that blonding has become easy on the hair and scalp, easy on the pocketbook and natural looking. Of these, being natural looking is the most important.

But natural or not, the desire for blondeness is centuries old. Even in Roman times, blonde hair was the fashion. The blonder the woman, the more she was admired.

And for those Roman women who weren't fair-haired, there were wigs made from Teutonic or British hair. According to Ovid, those blonde wigs were worth their weight in gold. The Britons and Germans, knowing this, lightened their hair with a kind of soap made of goat's tallow and beechwood ashes.

By the Middle Ages, fair hair was so popular that Vincent de Beauvais, an author of the time, provided "recipes" for bleaching hair in a book called *Speculum Naturalae.*

Through the ages women the world over have found methods for blonding. In Venice the women basked in the rays of the sun believing it would make their hair gold, and at night they sat in the moonlight because they believed that was the way to turn their hair strawberry blonde. In France women once bleached their hair with a preparation of dried onion skins.

Fortunately the methods have changed.

In the 1930's and 1940's, when blonding was first available in beauty salons, the process meant hours of sitting and waiting, and even then results were uncertain.

Today a woman can change her hair color quickly and with predictable results. The questions today are not how long and how much, but rather what color and what method.

There's nothing like a personal consulation to determine your correct color and look, but short of that, here are the kinds of questions you might ask, and here is the right man to answer them.

He is Dominic Durastanti, a color expert who ran a fine salon in Shaker Heights, Ohio, and has colored the heads of thousands of women over the past thirty years.

How can you tell if a woman should color her hair?
If she wears makeup, she should color her hair.

That means everybody, or practically everybody. Be more specific.
What I'm saying is that any woman who knows enough to use makeup to give her looks a lift is smart enough to know that the right hair color will give her still more of a lift.

When a woman comes to you for a consultation, what's the first thing you notice before you decide on the color?
I look at her skin tone. That's the most important consideration, and if she has olive skin, I tell her she should not go blonde. If I make an olive-complexioned woman blonde, her skin will look unnatural.

Is natural the most important thing?
Absolutely. I think all hair color should be so natural you don't even know you're seeing it. All you should see is a woman who looks terrific, but you're not sure just what single feature is outstanding.

Suppose a young girl wants color. What do you advise?
To me young girl means teenager. I think teenagers should add a sun-kissed look to their hair, maybe a little hair painting, but nothing more. You know, there are more than twenty-five different hair colors in a young woman's hair. Sometimes we can do more with a cut to bring out color, and many times I'll suggest that a woman change her hair style to play up the

natural differences in color. That long, draggy look that teenagers wore for years didn't do much to dramatize the hair color.

When do you think women should really start to use color?
For most women the hair begins to age at twenty-five. Aging is that graying, fading, dull look. Since the hair provides the frame for the face, the whole look begins to change when the hair ages. I think aging hair makes a woman look as old as wrinkles. So at twenty-five every woman should get a color analysis.

And color makes the face look younger?
The right color makes a woman look younger, the wrong color adds years.

Now we're back at the beginning. How does a woman tell right from wrong?
I'm giving you very general rules, but I believe that a woman under forty with olive skin and dark hair should add some brown streaks that blend in with her look and add light around the face.

And what about a woman who's forty and whose hair is gray?
The woman whose hair was dark will look different at forty, and often she can go lighter because her skin tone will change. But even if her skin still has olive overtones, she should lighten her hair—go chestnut or some warm brown because if she covers her gray with a dark color, she'll find that the dark hair accentuates lines and wrinkles.

Don't you ever darken hair?
Yes. If the woman is young and has a sort of nondescript brown hair and wants a more positive, darker color.

Do many women do this?

No. I'd say that less than ten percent of all the women who get color at our salon go darker.

Suppose a woman analyzes her skin tone, decides she can be a blonde. What do you look for next?
The best way is to make her a natural-looking blonde. That means I never try to give her a flat color.

What's flat color?
An overall one-color look.

What's the best blonde look?
Dimensional color, the look of a child's hair. To see what I mean, look at the hair of a child from six to ten years of age. You'll see that the hair is never the same shade from the root to the end, never a solid color.

But how can you use a childlike color on an older woman? Isn't that incongruous?
No, because it's based on her own look and color, but it takes skill to find the precise color. Very few women can find the color by themselves the first time. One of the reasons women are unhappy with hair color is that they try it once at home and don't like the look they get.

What do you advise?
Obviously, I recommend getting the hair colored first in a quality salon that's known for its fine colorists. I think the best investment a woman can make is to put herself in the hands of a qualified professional the first time.

Otherwise?
Otherwise she might go too dark, get a solid color that's hard looking, old, unnatural and too severe.

Isn't this very expensive?
Not as expensive as making a mistake at home.

What do you think about drastic change?

I think your hair color has to go with your total look, your life style, your feeling about yourself. I love it when I color a woman's hair and I see her look at herself and smile. You have to remember that no one looks at you the way you look at yourself. A woman sees every hair on her head; nobody else does. You're more critical of yourself than other people are of you. After all, they don't look at you as anxiously as you see yourself.

Any warnings before a woman colors?

Remember that the first time even a hairdresser may not get the precise color you want; it takes time to know just how your hair "grabs" color. But all color when done by an expert can be corrected quickly—so relax and become the blonde you ought to be.

Important Facts About Hair

Before you attempt to color your hair, however, you should know basic hair facts so you can read labels intelligently and talk knowledgeably with hair professionals.

All hair is made up of a protein called keratin, the same protein our nails are made of. Because the hair and nails were originally meant to protect our bodies, they are quite resistant to most environmental factors.

Water, for example, won't damage the hair. (This is important to remember when you wonder about the dangers of too much shampooing.)

What can hurt the hair?

Prolonged exposure to ultraviolet light (strong sunshine, for instance) will weaken and bleach the hair and make it brittle.

You can also hurt the hair by using strong alkalis. Look carefully at the ingredients labeling on hair-relaxing products, for many of them have strong alkalis.

Only a woman who has waited for a haircut to grow out can realize the frustration of slow-growing hair. But while it may seem that one's hair is taking forever to reach a desired length, actually all hair grows at the rate of about 6 inches a year.

There are variations, of course. A hair fiber is formed within a follicle and extruded from it at the rate of one sixty-fourth of an inch per day or about one-half inch per month or six inches per year, but this may vary from person to person depending on the individual's reaction to season, nutrition, general health and age.

Although the thickness of hair varies as well as the rate of growth, a full head of hair is considered to contain 100,000 hair fibers.

Each hair fiber is composed of a core containing long, narrow cells called the cortex. Covering the cortex is an outer layer of flat, overlapping scale cells (somewhat like fish scales), and this is the hair's protective shield. It protects against plain old mechanical wear: abrasion by combing and brushing, pillows, hats, practically anything you can think of.

As hair emerges from the follicle, it has six to eight layers of scales. With time the outer layers wear out, the inner ones become exposed, and about 18 inches down the shaft, or about the time the hair is three years old, there are only three or four layers left.

That's why as hair gets longer it gets weaker. There simply isn't as much protection for the ends of longer hair.

But when you see split ends and breakage in your hair that's less than 18 inches long, that may be a signal that you haven't been good to your hair.

Hair that's badly treated will lose its scales much more rapidly and have only one or two layers left by the time it's two years old, or 12 inches long.

The greatest damage we do to our hair is to over-brush, overcomb, sit in the direct sun, and permit water damage from chlorination. So to protect the hair don't brush or comb too frequently, stay out of the sun and always wear a bathing cap when you swim in chlorinated water.

Yet no matter what kind of care you take of your hair, no one's hair will grow indefinitely. Each hair follicle goes through an active stage that lasts three to four years, and then it rests for several months before producing hair again. And when the rest period begins, the hair from that follicle is shed.

That means that a loss of 50 to 100 hair fibers a day is normal and inevitable.

Don't panic when you see hair in your brush or comb. It's normal, and normal is different for every person.

But if your hair loss really does seem excessive, check with a doctor. There are many reasons for hair loss, some of which may be environmental, nutritional or related to your general health or heredity.

Dr. George J. Berakha has noted that natural blondes tend to have drier scalps than brunettes, and blonde hair is finer, more brittle and more delicate and, therefore, more easily damaged or lost.

But no doctor knows precisely why hair gets gray. What we do know is that color, blonde and otherwise, is determined by the amount, size and shape of the melanin particles which are in the keratin of the cortical cells. (Red hair, however, is determined by a different substance called phaemelanin.) The hair gets gray when the follicles stop producing pigment, but we don't know why they stop producing it, nor do we know how to prevent that from happening.

There is much we do know about hair care, however, and *Blonde Beautiful Blonde* has developed guidelines for healthy hair.

60

General Hair Care

• *Wash your hair as often as it needs.* For some people with generous oil, once a day may be necessary. If your scalp is dry and your hair brittle, wash less frequently.

The day's relative humidity and the amount of steam heat in your home or office influence the number of times a week, or times a day, that you should wash your hair. And by the same token, your hair will behave differently in Florida than it will in Maine. To avoid damage to your hair, a simple rule to follow is: the more often you wash your hair, the quicker you take the soap off. Daily washing should mean leaving the soap on a matter of seconds. Soap and rinse. Rubbing does no good. Scrubbing of your scalp may feel great, but it isn't great for your hair. An overdose of soap does damage your hair.

• *Eat the right foods related to hair health.* Gelatin is a protein that is beneficial to the hair. Vitamin B in the form of Brewer's yeast tablets is definitely healthy for your hair. That's the word from Philip Kingsley whose Trichological Center in New York solves the hair problems of royalty, movie stars—and working men and women.

• *Comb hair, but don't brush a lot.* Brushing breaks the hair. The worst damage done to hair is caused by excessive brushing and teasing. More on this in the next section.

• *Use a conditioner always, on all types of hair,* to make the hair shinier, easier to style and softer to touch. Use lots of moisturizing conditioner in the winter because steam heat and the cold air of the Northeast dry the hair. Use a detangler or creme rinse on long, wet hair to help prevent split ends and breakage when you brush. Once a month take time to give your hair a treatment with a deep-penetrating conditioner; use a cap and heat. This can be done at home or in a salon. Make your conditioner work harder by applying before exercising. Wrap the head in a terry towel. Body heat during exercise will increase the results of the conditioner, and the towel will protect your hair from the elements.

• *Add curl by wetting the hair and setting it in rollers.* Apply just enough tension to the hair to roll it smoothly. Excessive tension stretches the hair, making it progressively weaker.

• *Never use brush rollers, and never roll too tight.*

• *Use a drier only until the hair is damp dry, not bone dry.* More on this later, too.

• *Stay out of the sun because sun bleaches, oxidizes and eventually makes hair dry and brittle.* Be careful of saltwater and chlorinated water when you swim. Wear a cap or rinse the hair with fresh water immediately after swimming.

• *If you go into the sun, cover your hair.* Sun bleaches and fades the color. It can even make hair dry and brittle.

• *Always comb wet hair with a large-tooth comb—* whether or not the hair is color-treated. Every time you feel a slight tug or encounter a tangle and just plow through it, you are either breaking off or weakening some particular hair on your head. If it doesn't break off then, it will be weaker than the other hairs on your head that have not been overstretched by combing or brushing. It will break off sooner than the rest.

A good test for determining whether your hair is suffering from excess breakage is to section off a small strand of hair and feel how thick that section is at the roots. Slide your fingers down the strand and see if you have the same thickness at the ends. If the hair thins out part way down and finishes off in a very few hairs at the end, you are mistreating your hair. What's more, you are encouraging more breakage by leaving it in that state. The quick remedy for the condition is to cut your hair short enough to be rid of most of the thin ends.

Brushes and Combs

Remember when you thought you needed a lot of firm brushing for healthy hair?

Well, nobody seems to think so anymore.

Nowadays brushing is done gently to style your hair, remove dust and distribute oils.

What brush should you buy?

There's no one brush that's exactly right for all women all the time. You should pick your brush according to your hair style.

But regardless of brush shape, observe these suggestions:

• Make sure your brush has bristles that can smooth your hair without damaging. Most beauty authorities think that natural, round-tipped, wild boar bristles give the most control.

• If you have medium-to-coarse hair use a brush with the stiffer dark boar's bristle.

• If you have fine, delicate hair (definitely the blonde type), use the pale-bristle brushes because they're gentler on the hair.

Today you need a wardrobe of brushes to keep your hair in style. If you wear your hair short, use a narrow, flat-bristle brush. Medium-to-long hair, use a brush that is slightly rounded and lets you turn your hair up or under.

To handle thick hair, try a curved bristle, rubber-base brush.

The rounder the better is what I find for blow-drying. And for hair around the face, hair that you may want to turn up and curl gently, use a small, long, rounded brush with bristles all around. Roll the hair gently, and blow.

Combs should not dig the scalp; the best ones are the curved ones with the rubber-tipped teeth. For after shampooing, you should comb the hair with a big-tooth comb so that the hair is pulled as little as possible. Remember that wet hair (especially hair that's colored) is easily damaged by reckless combing.

Now one added tip: to hold your look after you've combed and brushed it into place, try one of the new non-aerosol hair sprays. And I think the best and most natural way to use it is to spray your brush, then stroke your hair. Pretty!

Guides to Getting a Good Haircut

Blonde isn't only in the color; it's in the cut.
And you've got to have the cut for blonde.
Since it's impossible to reverse a haircut you don't like, here are some tips *before* you make an appointment for a cut.

1. Look at your friends, decide whose haircut you most like (and whose cut is closest to the one you want), and ask for the name of the person who cut her hair.
2. Visit the shops of good stylists the same way you would visit a surgeon before you schedule the operation.
3. Have a consultation with the stylist, and see what he or she suggests for you. Bring along pictures of cuts you like.
4. Watch the stylist cut someone's hair. A good stylist never cuts hair only while the customer sits. Make sure the woman whose hair is being cut *stands* at some point during the procedure so the stylist can

see the total look of the cut.

5. Never go to a shop known for a specific cut. Chances are you'll come out looking like everyone else—a haircut on a face instead of a face with a haircut that flatters it.
6. Don't let anyone talk you into a cut you don't think you want. It's always better to cut less the first time and go back a second time. It may be more expensive in terms of time and money, but you'll feel a lot better about what you're doing.
7. Avoid trends. If the whole world is short and layered, remember that your streaks will look more like stripes than streaks if you cut and layer your hair.
8. Do your coloring after your cutting—that way your new waves and lines can be highlighted.
9. Ask prices in advance.

Hair Appliances and Their Use

Don't let anyone kid you.

When you color your hair, you get the advantage of what color does for you plus the advantage of hair that is often fuller and in better condition.

But hair that is colored requires special care to avoid breakage and other damage. And misuse of appliances is one of the ways to hurt any hair, colored or natural. So be sure you use appliances correctly.

And because you're blonde, you want to be especially careful to avoid hair damage because blonde hair tends to be more fragile.

Now for some questions and answers about the best way to use appliances.

Will an instant hairsetter (electric rollers) work on every kind of hair?

Definitely.

But for best results, use according to your hair texture:

- Oily or thick hair: leave the rollers on an extra minute or two.
- Dry hair: rub a gentle moisturizing hairdressing on the ends of your hair before using.
- Fine and thin hair: use a good conditioner for extra body.

If my hair is very dry, should I use the hairsetter less often?

Women with very dry hair should use a conditioning mist hairsetter because it can be used as often as you want. These three-way hairsetters are good because they give you conditioning mist, water mist and a regular set.

Is there a special way to roll the hair on electric rollers?

It's very important to wind the hair evenly for total heat penetration, because the roller's heat produces the set.

Make sure the ends of the hair are perfectly smooth around the roller.

Roll carefully but firmly until the roller touches your head (gently, not tightly).

When you're ready to unwind, do it slowly and gently. Then let the hair cool a minute or two before you comb it into a soft style.

How do I know which size rollers to use?

- Jumbo rollers are for body and gentle wave movement.
- Large rollers give the hair body and more clearly defined waves.
- Medium rollers are for firmer curls and deep wave patterns (this is recommended for long hair).
- Small rollers give you very firm curls, and should be used on tendrils and that hard-to-curl, back-of-the-neck area.

I go crazy every time I look for a hair drier. There are so many different kinds. Which is best?

The drying capability of a drier is determined by the rate of air movement (velocity) as well as wattage (heat). So don't make your choice on wattage alone.

The best drier is one that gives you several different heat/air movement settings.

The amount of wattage you need is determined by your own individual hair type and the look you want to achieve.

For example, long thick hair needs the highest wattage to reduce drying time. Short, thin hair doesn't need as much power.

If you style your hair with combs or brushes as you dry it, medium or low wattage should be used. Hairdressers see a lot of breakage—particularly in the back where women tend to use high heat and stretch the hair as they reach back to dry it.

The thing to remember is that you must treat your hair gently, especially if it's dry or damaged. And if you select a drier with separate controls for wattage and air movement, you can combine low wattage with high air movement.

What's the correct way to use a hand-held drier?

Use the highest heat to finger-dry very wet hair quickly.

Then switch to medium or low heat to dry and style damp hair.

Any other features that are important?

Yes. Look for a wide-angle nozzle. This provides greater air flow throughout the hair so you can easily finger-push curly locks into shape.

And you'll probably be happiest with a drier that's compact, lightweight and (if you travel abroad) has dual voltage.

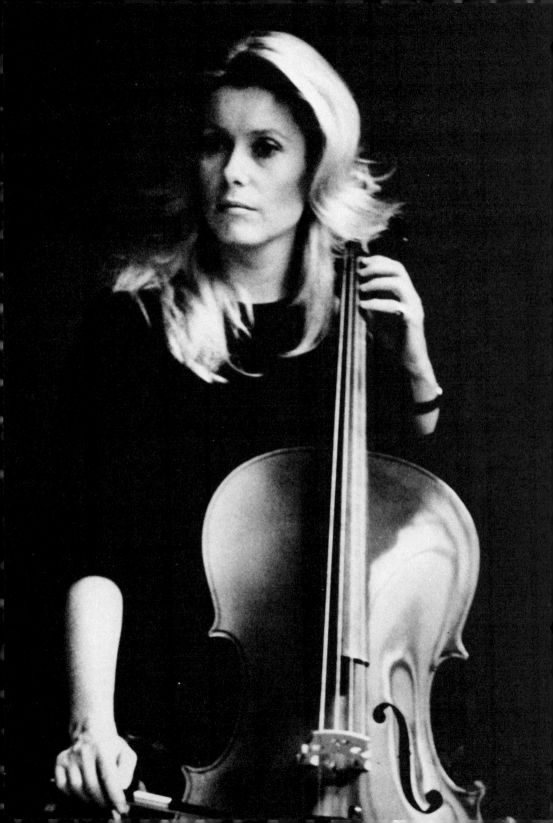

That Fabulous Face

"I can take a woman
and make her beautiful
for one picture,
but it takes more
than a makeup artist
to make her truly beautiful."

Sara McBandy

Catherine Deneuve: a cool, sophisticated blonde look

No one would disagree with makeup artist Sara McBandy, least of all the women who have made themselves over as blondes. Almost all women who become blonde see their blondeness as a first step and a stimulus for the next step. Blonding is the beginning of a change in self-image and personality.

For most women, the next "easy" step ("easy" meaning "instant") in a makeover is new makeup. When a woman changes her hair color, she must also change her makeup. Just as hair is colored lighter as a woman gets older, so should her makeup go lighter.

As we've said before, hair color must be keyed to complexion tones.

In the same way, *the shades of your makeup must be determined by skin tones, not by hair color or the color of the clothes.*

The Scandinavian Blonde Look works best on fair-skinned, blue-eyed women because the hair color really tends more toward the sunny yellow hues.

The California Look can range from medium to very, very light blonde and has rich, warm brown or amber tones and can therefore be worn by women with hazel eyes and skin tones deeper than the Scandinavian Blonde's.

The New York Blonde Look tends toward the deeper ash blonde shades, and is perfect for women with brown or green eyes and ruddier complexions, because a good ash blonde can tone down the ruddiness.

The Palm Beach Blonde Look is the coolest of all blondes, and ash-blonde hair shades are sensational on her porcelainlike skin, regardless of eye color.

The Newport Blonde Look is gray- or blue-eyed and against her rugged good looks and darker complexion go the darker blonde colors.

Now to the specifics.

Your Skin

Before thinking about makeup, there are certain things you must consider about the skin itself. Natural blondes' skin is generally more fragile, tends more to dryness and shows the effects of aging earlier (that's a euphemism for *wrinkles*).

So how do you take care of such delicate skin?

First, stay out of the sun. In addition to the danger of cancer caused by overexposure to the sun's rays, there's the cosmetic damage the sun does. Look at a woman in her forties who's spent her youth on a chaise in the sun. Then look at her friend who's been in the next chaise, protected by a hat, glasses, scarves and a sun screen. Of course, we all know the skin ages, but you can work to keep your skin looking soft and firm, and the first rule is—no sunning.

Two other rules are no smoking and only limited drinking. Tobacco and alcohol (aside from what they do to the inside of your body) also harm the outside because they affect the good circulation necessary to a healthy glow.

Another rule (and this is the hardest to follow) is *avoid tension.* I haven't found how to avoid tension in this life, but I do know that when I'm upset, tense and anxious, my skin doesn't look healthy. Conversely, when I feel happiest, my skin seems to glow. But for most of us tension isn't something we can easily remove from our lives.

And—especially if you're under thirty—the less makeup, the more natural you'll look. But no matter your age, don't overlook the moisturizer.

Moisturizing

There are dermatologists who believe that moisturizers are unnecessary, but the ones who think that are always men. I think moisturizing makes a big difference in the looks and feel of any skin that tends toward dryness. If you can feel tautness in your cheeks or see flaking, use a moisturizer morning and night. The makeup people I know, men and women, all use it. Moisturizers—the creams—should be applied during the day. At night, after cleaning, the skin is kept supple with an oil rather than a cream moisturizer. The secret of night oil is to apply sparingly, otherwise you may crawl into bed resembling a human banana peel.

Use eye cream under the eyes and on the lids, and with upward strokes apply a throat cream.

Then, if you can afford it, get a professional facial two or three times a year. The professional gives your skin a light peel to remove dead cells, and that makes the skin feel fresh and removes the dull gray look of some complexions.

There is no specific time when one must have a facial, but it can lift the spirits and make you feel good about yourself, particularly at the time of the changing of the seasons.

Cleansing

Contrary to popular belief, soap and water don't hurt your skin. In fact, soap and water clean your skin better than anything else. And water is important to keep your skin moisturized. It's the water, not the creams, that give your skin its moisture. The purpose of creams is to trap the water, hold it in and help your skin stay fresher longer.

To cleanse your face at night, use cold cream (I like it better than liquid makeup removers). Then wash the face with a mild superfatted soap (check the label) to get rid of all the grease and really clean the pores. Next splash with water to add moisture to the skin. Follow with a gentle toweling and night oil.

In addition, use a facial masque regularly. Good ones are available at any cosmetics counter, but be sure you find one that is right for your skin type. For blondes this generally means a non-drying rose masque because it is formulated for drier skins. A masque takes about twenty minutes and should be a part of a weekly beauty regimen.

Review:
Everything Your Face Needs

Moisturizer (use all day every day)
Cleansing cream
Liquid freshener
Mild soap
Night oil
Eye cream
Throat cream
Facial masque

All should be no-fragrance products.

Makeup

If you follow a good diet, exercise regularly, approach life with tranquillity, get plenty of rest and have a comfortable business and pleasant social life—well, you may never need any makeup at all.

Because there are no cosmetics that can take the place of any of those "natural cosmetics."

But since most of us go stumbling and bumbling through life, missing here and there, cosmetics are important to enhance our looks and to protect our skin from harmful things around us.

This book isn't written to extol any cosmetic product. Pick your own brands. Along the way, however, we'll give you some tips to help in the selection.

And remember—less is more.

Deborah Raffin, the blonde actress, made her hair darker for her role as Brooke Hayward in "Haywire." "I found that as a brunette I could use a lot more makeup than I could as a blonde," she said. "I never realized until then how subtle the makeup for a blonde must be in order to keep from looking overly painted."

Good words for all blondes.

In the order in which it should be applied, here's the daytime makeup you'll need.

Moisturizer (you've read about that on the preceding pages)
Foundation
Concealer
Eye makeup (shadows, liners, mascaras)
Blusher
Face powder
Lipstick: glosses and pencils

Foundation

After using moisturizer, apply a foundation.

The foundation is the key to a good makeup job because it's the canvas on which you'll create the face you want.

Stay with ivory or beige tones for your foundation. Don't try to emulate a suntan with a dark foundation; it only looks strange to see the makeup mark end somewhere around the neck or chin.

If you're suntanned, you may not even need a foundation (but don't you remember? Blondes are supposed to stay out of the sun).

The purpose of your foundation is to
1. Give the skin a smooth look.
2. Even the color of the face (more bare faces have various skin colors, everything from sallow blotches to patches of ruddiness).

3. Protect the skin from heat, sun and cold.

4. Provide a base for additional cosmetics.

Should you use a water- or oil-based cosmetic?

It really doesn't make much difference. What does matter is the amount you use. Don't overuse any product. More isn't better. The important thing is to keep a sheer film on your face, not a heavy mask. The heavy mask hides a young complexion and tends to settle in the lines and stay on top of drier, older skin.

To apply liquid makeup, pour a little into the palm of your hand and add a couple of drops of your moisturizer. Use your finger to blend, then apply dots to the forehead, cheeks and chin. Now with your fingers, blend out to the hairline and down to the chin. (Sara McBandy taught me this trick; she claims that blending in the hand makes the foundation go on better, and as far as I can see, she's right.) If you use a cake makeup, apply it with a damp sponge—very lightly.

A Word About Contouring

There are some makeup artists who can give you a totally different look with contouring. Contouring, as you know, is the subtle use of shadows and highlights to minimize deficiencies and maximize potential.

In the hands of an expert (Way Bandy once worked with me and did my makeup, and I couldn't believe I was the same person who'd walked into that room an hour earlier)—well, in the hands of an expert, contouring is an art to be admired.

But most of us are awkward. Applying eye makeup is enough of a chore, in terms of both time and ability, without adding any more challenges.

My own advice is to make the most of your own good features in other ways and leave the contouring to the experts. After all, with the power of blonde, you can afford it.

Concealer

Think that foundation alone is a concealer?

Not if you have dark circles under your eyes (all the time, not just when you stay out late or eat or drink unwisely), an occasional blemish or shadows on the forehead or around the nose.

To minimize or "light out," use a concealer.

Concealers come in stick form and in cream form. Some manufacturers tell you to use them before foundation, but I have always found that with a light hand, they work better after the foundation.

Choose a concealer that is one shade lighter than your foundation. Then, even if it's a stick, pat it onto the area to be treated. Spread it by dotting with your fingers. No rubbing, please.

Eye Makeup

Some do's and don'ts about the color of the eye makeup you choose:

1. No blonde *ever ever ever* should use blue or green eye shadow. It's just too obvious, even for Type A Blondes at the hottest disco in town.
2. If you have brown eyes, stay with the rust and plum tones.
3. If you have blue eyes, use the lavender shades, amethyst, heather.
4. If you have hazel eyes, stay with sandy pink, toast, grays.
5. If you have green eyes, your best colors are heather and rose.
6. If you have shaggy brows, let an expert shape them. The first time it's important to have a professional show you exactly where your brow should

be, and then you can follow the line by plucking the strays as they grow in.

For your eye makeup you'll need—
Eye shadow
Eyeliner pencils
Eye-makeup brushes
Eyelash curler
Mascara

Some experts use pencils for everything. Personally, I like the cake eye shadow, which is applied with a sponge.

To apply, find the brow bone (yes, it's there), and follow that line gently. Smudge the color with a brush or the sponge applicator.

Next comes a soft pencil eyeliner.

Dot the lash area around the eye with the pencil (don't forget the outside corner), and then with a small brush, smudge the look that you carry out toward your hairline.

Colors: black, brown, navy (I especially like the new Kohl pencils for underlining).

Now take your eyelash curler.

Press and hold while you count to 20.

And then apply mascara. Twice.

For an extra touch to make eyes look bigger, add navy or green liner (pencil) inside the lower lid. Lavender works magic, too.

Be sure to use your foundation on eyelids—it holds makeup better. But blot it before adding eye shadow; it will hold still better.

And if you want to use less mascara, or eliminate it altogether, dye your eyelashes. But not at home, never at home. That is a job for professionals.

Blusher

Blushers are always right for every face.

The amount and color you use depends on your skin tone and life style.

To apply a blusher, with your fingers feel the cheek bone on the side of your face. Apply blusher to the spot on the bone just under the middle of the eye, and carry the color out along the bone to the hairline.

Used this way, the blusher emphasizes your eyes.

Face Powder

A lot of women don't use it at all.

Some use baby powder.

My preference is a plain translucent powder.

With a clean cotton puff, dot the area on the forehead above the nose, then the nose and the chin.

Blend with a big brush.

Don't powder the whole face—just the center from the area above the nose to the chin. Don't ever powder the cheeks; don't powder away your healthy glow.

Lipstick and Glosses

There are two lip looks that detract from your blondeness: the undone lip and the overdone lip.

Never leave the lips nude. They look parched, dry.

But don't err on the side of greasy kid stuff. The look of overaccented lips is equally unappealing.

Even if you're at home where no one will see you, put something on your lips to protect them.

Here's the best way to create a pretty mouth:

Outline with a pencil.

Fill in with lipstick (apply with a brush at least the first time in the day), and don't blot.

Dot with gloss.

Night Moves

Natural, light-looking makeup is best for daytime.

But at night—pow! Experiment.

Night is a more daring time. Clothes are more seductive, conversation is more provocative and makeup should match the mood.

That's what a lot of women forget. Just as you change your clothes and your attitude, so should your makeup be different at night.

At night everything should go darker. Eyes, cheeks, lips.

Try more dramatic effects.

Put some pink lights in your bathroom or at your dressing table or wherever you put on makeup. I find that I get a subtler look under soft lights.

For the eyes, let them sparkle plenty. Don't be afraid to put color over color. Add glitter and shine with frosted and sparkle products.

And let the lips glisten. All you need is a touch of lip gloss in the center of the lips. Don't cover the whole lip. You're not out to win the greasy lips award.

Makeup Colors for Blondes

Whatever your reasons for choosing the shade of blonde you did, it will be for reasons of personality that you choose your makeup colors.

So *Blonde Beautiful Blonde* has created the Type A Blonde, the Type B Blonde and the Type C Blonde charts.

Like all rules, of course, they are made to be broken. For instance, a Type A woman may want a Type C look for a low-key meeting or business dinner. Conversely a Type B woman may want to take a fling with a Type A look one night. Go ahead. Have fun.

And get the look that's you today.

The Colors of Blonde

	Type A		Type B		Type C	
	Day	Night	Day	Night	Day	Night
The Look	Sophisticated	Dramatic	Town and Country	Elegant	Natural	Romantic
Foundation	Beige	Ivory	Natural beige	Yellow beige	Peachy beige	Sea shell, ivory, misty rose, beige
Blush	Rose	Red wine	Soft rose pink	Plum, dark rose	Pale peach, soft pink	Fragile rose, russet peach
Eye shadow	Clear lavender, brown	Gold, purple, dark fuchsia	Rust, heather	Mauve, dusty plum, amber brown	Sea pink, pale lilac, soft mauve	Deep lilac, pale amethyst, ginger rust
Eyeliner	Dark brown	Smoky plum, black	Brown	Navy blue, amethyst	Rust, ginger, pale aubergine	Soft lavender, shimmering brown
Mascara	Soft black	Dark plum, dark black	Brown/black	Navy blue, black	Russet, soft brown	Dark brown, soft black, lavender
Nail enamel	Plum	Red, wine	Clear mocha, rose	Deep mauve, deep rose, clear red	Sheer pink, soft peach, soft mocha	Deep rose, pale sepia
Fragrance	Y Red	Jungle Gardenia Opium Chloe	Miss Dior Caleche Partage	Joy Halston Amazon First Chamade Calandre	Diorissimo L'Air du Temps Mary McFadden	Pavlova Chanel No. 5 Nuit de Noel Chantilly
Lipstick	Dark rose, plum, raspberry	Currant, blue red, wine	Clear rose, soft chocolate, peach mocha	Deep rose, clear red	Pale pink, sand, soft peach	Light fuchsia, pale plum, pink

Plastic Surgery

But what if your face doesn't go with your blondeness?

Ever see a woman from the back and think she must be a vibrant, alive person only to have her turn around and you see a face that has aged faster than the rest of her?

That can happen to a blonde faster than any other woman.

Dr. James O. Stallings, a well-known plastic surgeon, says, "Blondes tend to age more rapidly. As sensitive as all humans are to sun, blondes are even more sensitive; their skin will wrinkle more easily, and for that reason will look older sooner."

So what's to be done?

Dr. Stallings believes there is nothing that can slow the aging process, no specific drug or cream or mumbo-jumbo.

The only answer to aging is to keep the aging process at a normal rate rather than an accelerated one.

How?

"With good skin care, proper diet and exercise," according to Dr. Stallings. He thinks "chin straps and facial exercises are a hoax. They accomplish nothing medically."

Nor do cosmetic products which are advertised to smooth lines in minutes. "All those products do," said Dr. George J. Berakha, the New York plastic surgeon, "is make the skin hold water. Because the skin is a little puffier, it looks as if the lines are not as deep."

For a real change, plastic surgery is the answer. "When a blonde has plastic surgery," Dr. Stallings said, "facelifts tend not to last quite as long. It's that thin skin. Blondes lose the elastic fibers of the skin more rapidly than brunettes.

"But now for the good news. Blondes tend to scar less. Their scars heal more favorably. I've never seen a keloid (raised scar) on a blonde."

Dr. Berakha also considers blondes better candidates for cosmetic surgery because "their thin, light skin leads to less conspicuous scars."

Obviously, a former brunette does not have blonde skin once she changes her hair color. So if you're a former brunette, you still have brunette skin traits, no matter what your hair color may be.

For facial-surgery patients, Dr. Berakha always analyzes the elements that make up the skin. He characterizes the typical blonde skin as fair, thin (not a lot of collagen, the protein that makes up the skin), dry (fewer sebaceous glands, which produce oil), with less elasticity and with lighter pigment (not a lot of melanin).

Dr. Berakha, like all skin specialists, cautions all patients to protect their skin from the sun because it causes earlier aging and can cause skin cancer.

In addition, he warns against hormone creams, which he calls "damaging." Said Dr. Berakha, "Hormones in creams can be absorbed into the body and have systemic effects. A woman should use hormone creams only if prescribed."

Do vitamin or protein creams have any special advantage?

No, according to Dr. Berakha.

He sympathizes with blondes, however, for they are more susceptible to laugh lines and tiny wrinkles, more prone to stretch marks because of their thin, dry skin.

But that same thin, dry skin is an advantage for rhinoplasty (nose operation), according to Dr. Berakha, "because the blonde's thinner skin adapts better to the new skeletal contour of the nose."

He also points out a blonde is a good candidate for

dermabrasion, the technique of smoothing the skin either when it has been damaged by acne scarring or is full of tiny wrinkles, such as the cracks around the lips. "The chief complication of this procedure is pigment change," Dr. Berakha cautions. "Therefore, the fairer blonde has less of a problem."

Time and again psychologists and other behavioral specialists have expressed the belief that blonding is a signal for total facial change, but Dr. Stallings doesn't agree.

"I talked to my colleagues around the country," he said, "and none of us feels that blondes come in for surgery any more often than women with other hair colors. It's about fifty-fifty, blondes and brunettes."

Dr. Berakha agrees with Dr. Stallings about facial surgery but not when it comes to body-sculpture surgery. "We see a high proportion of women who come in for breast surgery because after changing their hair color, they want to change their bodies."

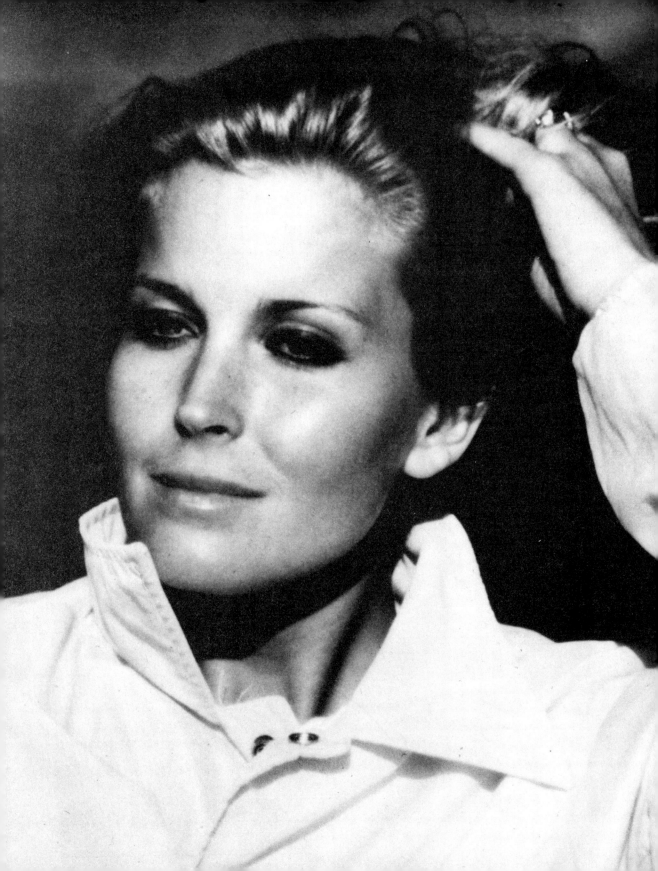

Getting To Your Kind of Blonde

*"Every human being
at one time or another
is concerned with physical appearance,
and wishes to change his own.
The most frequent change
undertaken by women,
and noticed by men,
is an alteration of hair color.
By far the most frequent change
is to a lighter shade."*

Roderic Gorney, M.D.

You don't have to be the cutest, youngest kid on the block to understand that blonde makes it on television.

Erma Bombeck, who's smarter and wittier and more sensible than half the women in the world and all the men in Washington, is now a blonde. A real blonde blonde. Look at her book jackets ten years ago. A brunette woman gazes thoughtfully at you. Today a snappy-looking blonde who seems a lot younger than the lady on the book jacket appears on TV. They are both Erma Bombeck.

Erma may talk about the dogs, the garbage and the septic tank. But evidently there are days when she is not cleaning the refrigerator and putting up Christmas decorations because our friend Erma has obviously been spending time with her hairdresser.

So if it's good enough for Cheryl Ladd and Erma Bombeck, maybe it's time you started to ask some questions—and get some answers.

How do you determine the hair color that is perfect for you?

The best way to see yourself in a color is to go to a department store and try on wigs. Find the shade you like on yourself, and then set out to duplicate it.

The surest way to learn how to get to your color is to go to the finest hair colorist in your city and get color applied professionally. I strongly recommend that any radical color change be supervised in a salon. After that, you can institute a program of home maintenance, but it's important to get to the right color first off and to take good care of your hair while doing it. If you're going more than a shade or two lighter than your natural color and you're doing it for the first time, then going to a salon is imperative for both your looks and your peace of mind. Be sure to ask the cost before any work is done, and shop the good salons.

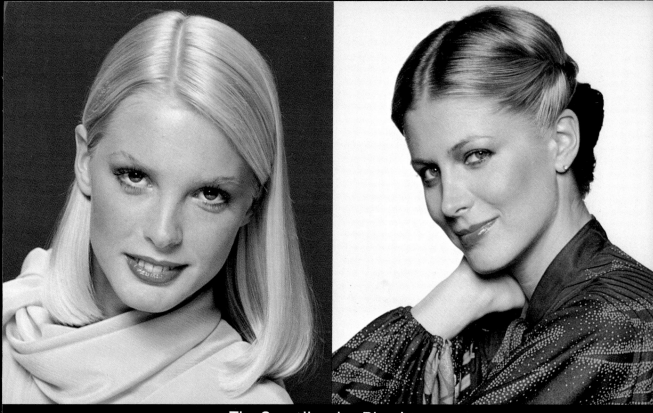

The Scandinavian Blonde

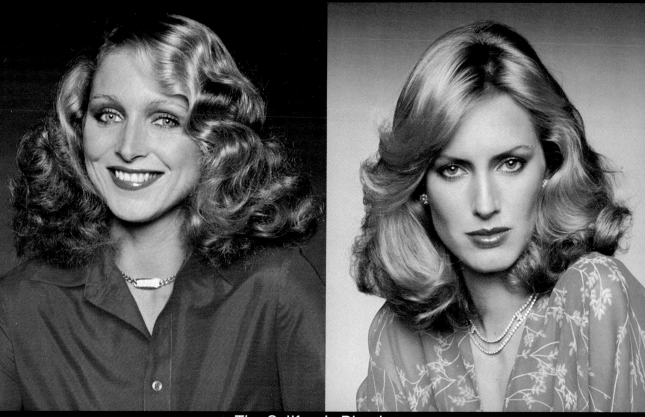

The California Blonde

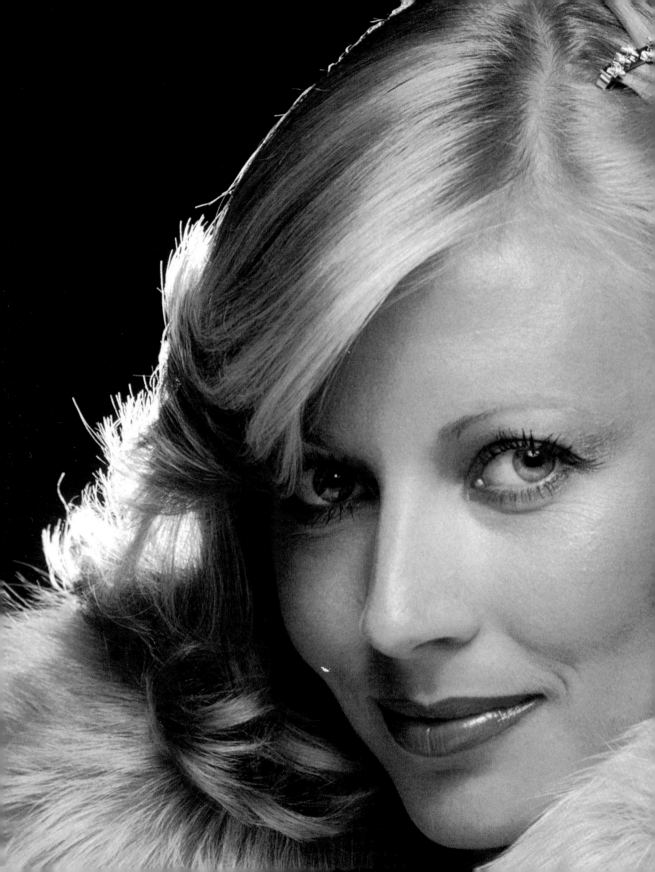

Hairstyles: Beautiful Blonde Looks

Fresh, sophisticated, enchanting.
Blondes can be all these,
and much of what a blonde
communicates about her looks
is through her hairstyle.
Here are some of the looks of
the 80's for blonde types.

The Palm Beach Blonde

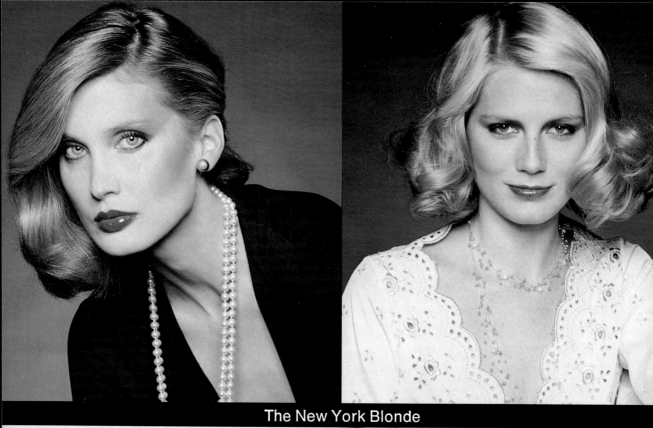

The New York Blonde

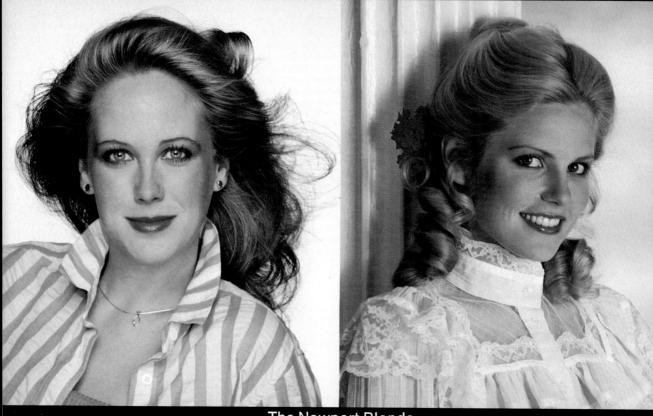

The Newport Blonde

How much will it cost?

The cost of color varies wildly.

You can color your hair at home with a variety of safe, easy-to-use products for less than $5.00. Or you can go to a famous salon (you read about them all the time in the fashion magazines) and spend as much as $100 to become blonde.

The cost of upkeep is equally disparate. It will cost just a few dollars to maintain colors at home every four to six weeks, and it could cost as much as $75 for a salon touch-up.

The differences in time should be understood, too.

Generally, the home methods are simpler and take less than an hour. A good salon will often take a whole morning or afternoon to work on your hair. Why such a difference? Because a salon checks its work as it progresses, and a good colorist adjusts the color to the way your hair shaft absorbs tint. So the professional may make changes as he or she goes along. The untrained home colorist isn't that kind of expert who can edit her work.

Is there a right kind of blonde for the texture and length of your hair?

"Absolutely," says Constance Hartnett, the color specialist at Louis-Guy D', the New York salon that specializes in cutting and coloring the hair of career women.

Frizzy, curly hair should be tinted with single-process color because, according to Constance, it will give the hair a silky, shiny look. Single-process gives the hair more depth, makes coarse hair look smoother.

Shoulder-length, straight hair can be streaked. For this woman there are fewer touch-up problems. Short, layered hair should never be streaked because it makes the woman look as if she has stripes. Streaked hair needs length because it has to have swing and movement to look right.

On the following pages are descriptions of the various kinds of hair color. They have been grouped according to the personality they fit, Type A, Type B or Type C Blondes with Type A referring to the more outgoing woman and Type C the more conservative.

Before you use any one of these colors, however, do—

1. Consult the shade chart to find the color best for you.
2. Take a patch test 24 hours before you use the color on your hair to determine whether there is sensitivity (or allergy) to a product. Paint a sample-size mixture on the skin (behind the ear or inside the elbow are two recommended places), and check 24 hours later to make sure there's no redness or breaking out of the skin.
3. Take a strand test before you apply color to your whole head. Oh, the problems women could avoid if they'd do this. Color a strand, and then look. Is it what you want? Too dark, too light? Even if you've been using the same product and the same color, it's important to take a strand test, because your own body chemistry—and certainly the condition of your hair—can vary the results from time to time.

Now, for your options and when and how to exercise them.

For highlights, subtle or dramatic:

Special Effects

Special effects take you closer to a blonde look without completely changing your hair color—or the way you see yourself. And it's important to remember in all hair color, that whatever you do will appear more dramatic, more unusual, more un-you to your eyes than anyone else's.

Most women find that after changing hair color—and nothing else—people look at them and say, "Something's different about you. I know. You lost five pounds."

Here are the ways to get some light-hearted blonde looks.

Hair Painting

This is the easiest of all the procedures. You start when your hair is dry, paint on streaks where you want them (generally around the face) and get the sense of finished hair with a little color added.

If you're doing it yourself (or your sister, mother or best friend is holding the brush), stay on the under-done side. You can always add more streaks later.

Frosting and Streaking

There are kits available for this, too. They come in two varieties.

The Cap Method: You tie a little cap that looks somewhat like a shower cap under your chin and pull selected strands through the cap with a crochet hook, then bleach them. The newest caps are color-marked to help you figure out the look you want. Coloring by cap is a little like painting by number.

Foil Wrap: You take the strands to be bleached, put the bleach on them, wrap them in foil, then take them out and presto! blonde streaks.

To see how a new color feels:

Temporary Color

Take a weekend when you're not going to face the world (or the most important people in your life) and do a little experimenting in your own bathroom. Then if you don't like what you get, simply shampoo it out the next day. That's the beauty of temporary color. It's not much more of a commitment than a new lipstick.

Temporary color works only on the outer circle of the hair and does not go into the cortex where the pigment is.

Unless your hair is already fairly light, you won't go truly blonde—you'll just see golden highlights—with a temporary color because *remember*: temporary rinses are coating the surface of the hair, not reaching the cortex.

But one thing about temporary color: Even if there's not an earthshaking difference to others, you'll look very different to yourself. And it's a light, bright, glad-to-be-me feeling.

To blend gray or enliven your natural blondness:

Semi-permanent Color

Since semi-permanent is such a contradiction in terms, you ought to know what it means in terms of application.

A semi-permanent hair color does a little of what a temporary color does and a little of what a permanent hair color does. That is, a semi-permanent permits *some* of the color to reach the cortex, whereas a temporary permits none. A semi-permanent color, however, cannot lighten the hair. It is used to blend gray in with your natural color.

Each time you wash the hair a little more of the color in the cortex reaches the cuticle (the outermost layer of the hair). After four or five washings, the color's gone—and you must reapply.

To transform your hair color—and you:

Permanent Single-Process Tints

This is what most of us use.

It's the easiest, most exciting, most convenient way to color. If I sound especially enthusiastic, it's that I've colored my own hair this way for years and find it natural looking and completely effective.

It's a one-process step which removes pigment and deposits color in the cortex of the hair shaft. At the same time, the hair is softened and plumped.

A permanent hair color can change your hair color or get rid of gray, but while it can make mousy hair lighter, it can't make a brunette blonde.

The best first usage is to go one shade lighter than your natural color. The color you get will be a combination of your own color and the added color. It's a real live look, not a dull, unnatural one.

Permanent shampoo-in tints are easy to apply. They come in a package with two bottles that you mix (one is a tint base, the other a developer). You apply it to dry hair, leave it on 20 minutes, then rinse out. You may or may not have to shampoo afterwards. So it is just one step.

The tint goes right to the cortex and stays.

You need new color only to keep up with new growth or because you get fading or color change from the environment (remember all those things such as sunlight, shampooing and chlorine that can change hair color).

To go from dark to light:

Double-Process Blonding

It's called double-process because it takes two steps.

And your first double-process application should probably be done in a salon.

What happens at a salon is that first you get a consultation (at a good salon this is the first step before any color is applied). Then if double-processing is indicated—

1. the hair is bleached to the desired shade of lightness;

2. then hair is colored to the desired shade of blonde.

This kind of blonding can also be maintained by a salon. One of the big problems in doing it at home is overlapping; that is, as you color again you inadvertently get more bleach on previously bleached hair. That can cause breakage. Of course, if you have a friend who's good with hair and is willing to help you, home can be the best place to color.

Double-process blonding is a commitment. You can't have dark roots, and you must take very good care of your hair (no overbrushing, overcombing, overshampooing or overexposing to heat, salt and elements).

This is the quickest, surest route to blonde. Real blonde. Not maybe, half-hearted blonde. But real live blonde.

Getting There: Experimenting

If this is your first experience in lightening your hair, don't go blonde overnight—particularly if you're a woman over 40 who's been a definite brunette all her adult life. Radical change makes husbands very unhappy, and children don't like that dramatic change in their mothers.

Instead move up one shade and experiment with color.

"It amazes me," says Constance Hartnett, "that women who will buy all kinds of fashion accessories won't buy more than one bottle of hair color to try at home. If you're going from brown to blonde, then you should begin down with the darker shade blondes, but experiment by adding a few drops of a lighter shade of blonde to the formula. On the other hand, if your final shade is to be a lighter blonde, you might add a few drops of the darker shade blonde. You may even want to mix half-darker shade and half-lighter shade. But I think you ought to understand that not many women can use a formula exactly the way it is in the bottle and get precisely the color they want the first time. You don't have to be afraid to mix—so long as you *use the same product. Don't ever mix two different brands.*

"You have to work for results, not pray for them," she said firmly.

Getting There: The Colors to Be

There isn't one kind of blonde any more than there's one kind of pickle. Now that you know your blonde personality type, you can fit type to look to method.

On the next pages, you'll find charts for blonding according to your present hair color, where you want your color to go and your life style.

So, first, decide whether you're a Type A, Type B or Type C Blonde. Remember the Type A woman is the more adventurous, the more outgoing. Type B is in tune with her times, fashionable, in season but not ahead of season. And Type C is more conservative. And pick your look—Scandinavian, California, New York, Palm Beach or Newport.

You'll see that more than one way is given to go from your own color to the blonde you want; we're attempting to cover the differences in your present color and the differences in shading in the color you want, so your own judgment obviously is very important here.

In all double-process blonding, you'll see that the first step requires the hair to be lightened to the necessary shade, with the second step giving you the desired final color. That's what double-process is all about: prelightening so the hair can accept the second step, which is color.

Getting There:
More Tips from a Pro

Constance thinks that home hair coloring is one of the great boons of womankind—certainly as important as the dishwasher, and almost as necessary as panty hose.

The first time I met Constance was at Louis-Guy D', the salon where she is resident color expect. "Will you color my hair?" I asked.

She inspected me carefully. "Who does it?"

"I do," I said meekly.

"Keep on doing it; I can't do better," she answered.

You see, Constance is honest and a believer in women doing what they can for themselves. That's why I asked her to give us home colorists some tips. Here they are:

• First, don't go too light. If you get red, brassy results, you've probably gone too light for your natural shade. Go down closer to your own real color.

• As for hennaing, don't be misled by its promises. Henna is a natural dye, but it's still a dye, so much so that once you henna your hair you can't change it back. Your only alternatives are cutting the hair or letting it grow out. With single- and double-process you have the option to recolor.

And it's not a conditioner. It can dry the hair and eventually ruin it if overused, so don't use henna more than three times a year.

Now for information on color selection and becoming your kind of blonde.

Colorings for the Type A Blonde

She exudes excitement by day and sizzles at night.
She's the woman with the drop-dead looks.
For her, men build bridges, write sonnets—even get married.

If your hair is—	Use—	To be—
Light brown or dark blonde (and your eyes are blue, gray or green)	Step 1: BORN BLONDE LIGHTENER Step 2: BORN BLONDE 360: Moonlit Mink *or* Step 1: NATURALLY BLONDE LIGHTENER Step 2: NATURALLY BLONDE TONER 411: Swedish Crystal 412: Autumn Ash	Medium-light blonde/ Scandinavian Look
	FROST AND TIP	Dramatically streaked/ California Look
Medium-light blonde (and regardless of eye color)	QUIET TOUCH	Dazzlingly highlighted/ Scandinavian or California Look
Salt and pepper (and your eyes are brown, gray, green or blue)	Step 1: BORN BLONDE LIGHTENER Step 2: BORN BLONDE 351: Silent Snow 352: Precious Platinum 353: Sweet Silver 354: Baby Blush 355: Blissfully Blonde 356: Innocent Ivory 357: Beautiful Beige 358: Winsome Wheat 359: Fair Fawn 361: Happy Honey 362: Sheer Strawberry *or* Step 1: NATURALLY BLONDE LIGHTENER Step 2: NATURALLY BLONDE TONER 401: Cool White 402: Platinum Blonde 404: Platinum Surf 405: Natural Pearl 406: Fair-Haired Blonde 407: Sunny Beige	Medium-light blonde/ New York, Palm Beach or Newport Look

If your hair is—	Use—	To be—

Medium-light blonde (and your eyes are brown, blue, green or gray)	408: Truly Beige
	409: Summer Haze
	410: Sifted Sand
	415: Softly Blonde
	
	*CLAIRESSE:
	200: Pale Blonde
	202: Pale Ash Blonde
	204: Light Ash Blonde
	*NICE AND EASY:
	  99: Palest Blonde
	100: Pale Blonde
	101: Pale Ash Blonde
	*MISS CLAIROL
	  CREME FORMULA:
	  16: Sunbeam Blonde
	  22: Nordic Blonde
	  30: Flaxen Blonde
	  40: Topaz
	*MISS CLAIROL
	  SHAMPOO FORMULA:
	16S: Sunbeam Blonde
	22S: Nordic Blonde
	30S: Flaxen Blonde
	40S: Topaz
	*BALSAM:
	600: Palest Blonde
	601: Light Ash Blonde
	*COLORSILK:
	9B: Pale Beige Blonde
	9A: Pale Ash Blonde
	8A: Light Ash Blonde
	*L'OREAL PREFERENCE
	9A: Light Ash Blonde
	9½A: Extra Lt. Ash Blonde
	9½BB: Extra Lt. Beige Blonde
		A brighter medium-light blonde/ California, New York Looks

Light brown or dark blonde (and your eyes are blue, gray or green)	Step 1: BORN BLONDE
	  LIGHTENER
	Step 2: BORN BLONDE
	360: Moonlit Mink
	or
	Step 1: NATURALLY BLONDE
	  LIGHTENER
	Step 2: NATURALLY BLONDE
	411: Swedish Crystal
	412: Autumn Ash
		Dark or medium blonde/ Scandinavian Look

Medium to light blonde (and your eyes are brown)	The same products recommended immediately preceding. This procedure is for the woman who wants to enrich the color of her hair when she sees color fading.	Dark blonde/ New York, Palm Beach or Newport Look

*These are all single-process colors.

Colorings for the Type B Blonde

She has wit and grace and style.

She's the woman who looks smart by day, appealing by night.

Men love her for the way she combines romance and common sense, which can—if you're lucky—be the same thing.

If your hair is—	Use—	To be—
Medium-light blonde (and your eyes are brown)	Step 1: NATURALLY BLONDE LIGHTENER Step 2: BORN BLONDE 401: Cool White 403: Platinum Breeze 404: Platinum Surf 405: Natural Pearl 406: Fair-Haired Blonde 407: Sunny Beige 408: Truly Beige 409: Summer Haze 410: Sifted Sand 415: Softly Blonde *or* Step 1: BORN BLONDE LIGHTENER Step 2: BORN BLONDE 351: Silent Snow 352: Precious Platinum 353: Sweet Silver 354: Baby Blush 355: Blissfully Blonde 356: Innocent Ivory 357: Beautiful Beige 358: Winsome Wheat 359: Fair Fawn 361: Happy Honey 362: Sheer Strawberry	A brighter medium-light blonde/ Scandinavian Look A brighter blonde/ California Look
Dark blonde	QUIET TOUCH	Softly highlighted/ California or Palm Beach Looks
Light brown (and your eyes are blue, gray or green)	*CLAIRESSE: 200: Pale Blonde 202: Pale Ash Blonde *NICE AND EASY: 99: Palest Blonde 100: Pale Blonde 101: Pale Ash Blonde *MISS CLAIROL CREME FORMULA: 16: Sunbeam Blonde 22: Nordic Blonde	Medium-light blonde/ California Look

If your hair is—	Use—	To be—

	30: Flaxen Blonde
	40: Topaz
	*MISS CLAIROL
	   SHAMPOO FORMULA:
	16S: Sunbeam Blonde
	22S: Nordic Blonde
	30S: Flaxen Blonde
	40S: Topaz
	*BALSAM:
	600: Palest Blonde
	601: Light Ash Blonde
	*COLORSILK:
	  9B: Pale Beige Blonde
	  9A: Pale Ash Blonde
	  8A: Light Ash Blonde
	*L'OREAL PREFERENCE:
	  9A: Light Ash Blonde
	9½A: Extra Lt. Ash Blonde
	9½BB: Extra Lt. Beige Blonde	

Salt and pepper
(and your eyes are
brown or gray)
	*CLAIRESSE:
	206: Golden Blonde
	208: Medium Ash Blonde
	*NICE AND EASY:
	105: Deep Golden Blonde
	106: Medium Ash Blonde
	*MISS CLAIROL
	   CREME FORMULA:
	  28: Autumn Mist
	  41: Golden Apricot
	*MISS CLAIROL
	   SHAMPOO FORMULA:
	28S: Autumn Mist
	41S: Golden Apricot
	*BALSAM:
	602: Ash Blonde
	604: Dark Blonde
	*COLORSILK:
	  7G: Golden Blonde
	  7A: Medium Ash Blonde
	*L'OREAL PREFERENCE:
	7½A: Medium Ash Blonde
	  8G: Golden Blonde
		Dark blonde/
		New York, Palm Beach
		or Newport Looks

Salt and pepper
(and your eyes are
blue or green)
	Step 1: BORN BLONDE
	  LIGHTENER
	Step 2: BORN BLONDE
	360: Moonlit Mink
	or
	Step 1: NATURALLY BLONDE
	  LIGHTENER
	Step 2: NATURALLY BLONDE
	411: Swedish Crystal
	412: Autumn Ash
		Medium blonde/
		Scandinavian or
		California Looks

*These are all single-process colors.

TYPE B (cont.)

If your hair is—	Use—	To be—

Salt and pepper
(and your eyes are blue)
	*CLAIRESSE:
	200: Pale Blonde
	202: Pale Ash Blonde
	204: Light Ash Blonde
	205: Soft Beige Blonde
	*NICE AND EASY:
	 99: Palest Blonde
	100: Pale Blonde
	101: Pale Ash Blonde
	102: Light Ash Blonde
	103: Light Beige Blonde
	104: Golden Blonde
	*MISS CLAIROL
	  CREME FORMULA:
	 16: Sunbeam Blonde
	 22: Nordic Blonde
	 27: Spring Honey
	 30: Flaxen Blonde
	 40: Topaz
	*MISS CLAIROL
	  SHAMPOO FORMULA:
	 16S: Sunbeam Blonde
	 22S: Nordic Blonde
	 27S: Spring Honey
	 30S: Flaxen Blonde
	 40S: Topaz
	*BALSAM:
	600: Palest Blonde
	601: Light Ash Blonde
	*COLORSILK:
	 9B: Pale Beige Blonde
	 9A: Pale Ash Blonde
	 8A: Light Ash Blonde
	 7G: Golden Blonde
	*L'OREAL PREFERENCE:
	9½BB: Extra Light Beige Blonde
	9½A: Extra Light Ash Blonde
	 9A: Light Ash Blonde
	 8G: Golden Blonde
		Medium-light blonde/
		New York or
		Palm Beach Looks

White (and your eyes are brown, gray or green)	*CLAIRESSE: 200: Pale Blonde 202: Pale Ash Blonde 204: Light Ash Blonde *NICE AND EASY: 99: Palest Blonde 100: Pale Blonde 101: Pale Ash Blonde 102: Light Ash Blonde 103: Light Beige Blonde 104: Golden Blonde *MISS CLAIROL CREME FORMULA:	Medium-light blonde/ New York or Palm Beach Looks

If your hair is—	Use—	To be—
	16: Sunbeam Blonde 22: Nordic Blonde 27: Spring Honey 30: Flaxen Blonde 40: Topaz *MISS CLAIROL SHAMPOO FORMULA: 16S: Sunbeam Blonde 22S: Nordic Blonde 27S: Spring Honey 30S: Flaxen Honey 40S: Topaz *BALSAM: 600: Palest Blonde 601: Light Ash Blonde *LOVING CARE: 72: Golden Blonde 73: Ash Blonde *LOVING CARE FOAM: 73F: Ash Blonde *HAPPINESS: 900: Ash Blonde *COLORSILK: 9B: Pale Beige Blonde 9A: Pale Ash Blonde 8A: Light Ash Blonde 7G: Golden Blonde *L'OREAL PREFERENCE: 9½BB: Extra Light Beige Blonde 9½ A: Extra Light Ash Blonde 9A: Light Ash Blonde 8G: Golden Blonde	

*These are all single-process colors.

Colorings for the Type C Blonde

She has the kind of casual good looks born to her face.
Color enhances what's there—but doesn't change it.
She's the woman every man is proud to call his wife.

If your hair is—	Use—	To be—

A medium-light blonde that's fading (and your eyes are blue or green)	*CLAIRESSE:
	205: Soft Beige Blonde
	206: Golden Blonde
	208: Medium Ash Blonde
	*NICE AND EASY:
	102: Light Ash Blonde
	103: Light Beige Blonde
	105: Deep Golden Blonde
	106: Medium Ash Blonde
	*MISS CLAIROL
	   CREME FORMULA:
	  26: Winter Wheat
	  28: Autumn Mist
	  41: Golden Apricot
	*MISS CLAIROL
	   SHAMPOO FORMULA:
	26S: Winter Wheat
	28S: Autumn Mist
	41S: Golden Apricot
	*BALSAM:
	602: Ash Blonde
	604: Dark Blonde
	*COLORSILK:
	  7G: Golden Blonde
	  7A: Medium Ash Blonde
	  8A: Light Ash Blonde
	  9B: Pale Beige Blonde
	*L'OREAL PREFERENCE:
	  8G: Golden Blonde
	  7½ A: Medium Ash Blonde
	  9A: Light Ash Blonde
	  9½BB: Extra Light Beige Blonde
		Darker blonde/
		Newport or
		Palm Beach Looks

Dark Blonde (and your eyes are blue, gray or green)	*CLAIRESSE: 200: Pale Blonde 202: Pale Ash Blonde 204: Light Ash Blonde *NICE AND EASY: 99: Palest Blonde 100: Pale Blonde 101: Pale Ash Blonde 102: Light Ash Blonde 104: Golden Blonde	Medium-light blonde/ Newport or California Looks

If your hair is—	Use—	To be—

Light brown
(and your eyes are brown,
gray, green or blue)
	*MISS CLAIROL
	  CREME FORMULA:
	  16: Sunbeam Blonde
	  22: Nordic Blonde
	  27: Spring Honey
	  30: Flaxen Blonde
	  40: Topaz
	*MISS CLAIROL
	  SHAMPOO FORMULA:
	  16S: Sunbeam Blonde
	  22S: Nordic Blonde
	  27S: Spring Honey
	  30S: Flaxen Blonde
	  40S: Topaz
	*BALSAM:
	  600: Palest Blonde
	  601: Light Ash Blonde
	*COLORSILK:
	  9B: Pale Beige Blonde
	  9A: Pale Ash Blonde
	  8A: Light Ash Blonde
	  7G: Golden Blonde
	*L'OREAL PREFERENCE:
	  9½BB: Extra Light Beige Blonde
	  9½A: Extra Light Ash Blonde
	  9A: Light Ash Blonde
	  8G: Golden Blonde
	
	*CLAIRESSE:
	  204: Light Ash Blonde
	  205: Soft Beige Blonde
	  206: Golden Blonde
	*NICE AND EASY:
	  101: Pale Ash Blonde
	  102: Light Ash Blonde
	  103: Light Beige Blonde
	  104: Golden Blonde
	*MISS CLAIROL
	  CREME FORMULA:
	  26: Winter Wheat
	  27: Spring Honey
	  41: Golden Apricot
	*MISS CLAIROL
	  SHAMPOO FORMULA:
	  26S: Winter Wheat
	  27S: Spring Honey
	  41S: Golden Apricot
	*BALSAM:
	  601: Light Ash Blonde
	  602: Ash Blonde
	*COLORSILK:
	  8A: Light Ash Blonde
	  7G: Golden Blonde
		Dark blonde/
		Newport Look

If your hair is—	Use—	To be—

Dark blonde
(and your eyes are brown)
	9A: Pale Ash Blonde
	9B: Pale Beige Blonde
	*L'OREAL PREFERENCE:
	9A: Light Ash Blonde
	8G: Golden Blonde
	9½A: Extra Light Ash Blonde
	9½BB: Extra Light Beige Blonde
	
	*CLAIRESSE:
	205: Soft Beige Blonde
	206: Golden Blonde
	208: Medium Ash Blonde
	*NICE AND EASY:
	102: Light Ash Blonde
	103: Light Beige Blonde
	105: Deep Golden Blonde
	106: Medium Ash Blonde
	*MISS CLAIROL
	  CREME FORMULA:
	26: Winter Wheat
	28: Autumn Mist
	41: Golden Apricot
	*MISS CLAIROL
	  SHAMPOO FORMULA:
	26S: Winter Wheat
	28S: Autumn Mist
	41S: Golden Apricot
	*BALSAM:
	602: Ash Blonde
	604: Dark Blonde
	*COLORSILK:
	7G: Golden Blonde
	7A: Medium Ash Blonde
	8A: Light Ash Blonde
	9B: Pale Beige Blonde
	*L'OREAL PREFERENCE:
	8G: Golden Blonde
	7½A: Medium Ash Blonde
	9A: Light Ash Blonde
	9½BB: Extra Light Beige Blonde
		A more golden blonde instead of "dirty" blonde/ California Look

Light brown (regardless of eye color)	GENTLE LIGHTS	Subtly highlighted/ New York or Newport Look
White (and your eyes are blue)	*CLAIRESSE: 206: Golden Blonde 208: Medium Ash Blonde *NICE AND EASY: 105: Deep Golden Blonde 106: Medium Ash Blonde *MISS CLAIROL CREME FORMULA:	Dark blonde/ Scandinavian, Palm Beach or Newport Looks

If you hair is—	Use—	To be—
	28: Autumn Mist 41: Golden Apricot *MISS CLAIROL SHAMPOO FORMULA: 28S: Autumn Mist 41S: Golden Apricot *BALSAM: 604: Dark Blonde *LOVING CARE: 72: Golden Blonde 73: Ash Blonde *LOVING CARE FOAM: 73F: Ash Blonde *HAPPINESS: 900: Ash Blonde *COLORSILK: 7G: Golden Blonde 7A: Medium Ash Blonde *L'OREAL PREFERENCE: 8G: Golden Blonde 7½A: Medium Ash Blonde	

*These are all single-process colors.

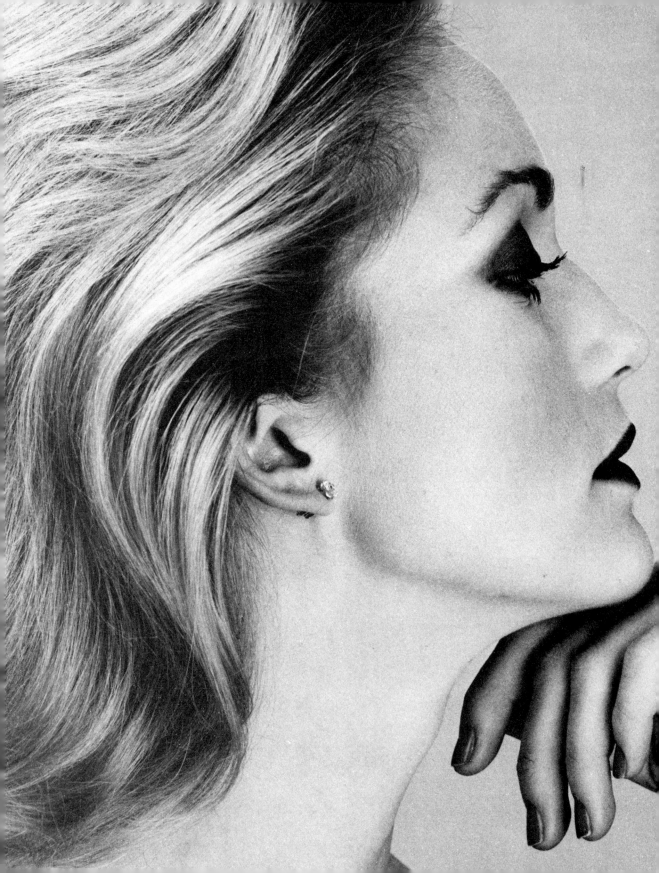

Questions, Questions, Questions,

"For the second marriage,
the woman is always blonde."

Rose Reti

Blonding requires a friend.

You just can't go blonde without talking to a friend. If you're lucky, the friend may be a professional hair colorist. But if you live in a city where it's difficult to find someone to answer all your questions or if your best friend doesn't know, it's good to realize that Clairol knows everything about blonding—and is waiting to tell.

A few years ago Clairol set up a toll-free number to be used anywhere in the United States. (In Continental United States, call 800-223-5800 or, in New York State, call collect 212-644-2990. Either number may be called Monday through Friday, from 8:30 a.m. to 8:00 p.m. EST.)

The service is part of the Consumer Relations Department, and the telephone consultants answer 24,000 inquiries each month. The consultants are all trained hair technicians, have completed a special course in hair and color work and are careful with their answers.

The question most frequently asked is—

How can I be a single-process blonde without red in my hair?

The colorists warn that the redness depends a lot on a woman's natural pigmentation. In general, the colorists advise first that a woman choose a blonde shade close to her own hair color. The ash-blonde shades are often the best. Color should not be kept on the hair any longer than advised in the instructions. (A lot of women think if you can get color in 20 minutes you can get better color in 30 minutes, but colors are timed for the instructions on the packages.)

The question most difficult to answer is—

What color should I be?

Consultants who don't see the way you look, stand, walk or talk have a difficult time prescribing shades over the phone. What they do is to try to help women decide just which shade of yellow they want in blonding by referring to colors of fruits and vegetables.

Terminology confuses women, and a constant question is—

What is meant by double-process?

Experts explain, this is coloring of hair by applying first a lightener and then a toner. The lightener takes the red out of the hair, and the toner gives it a delicate blonde shade.

The most concerned callers are the women who say—

I have a new boyfriend. He doesn't know I'm not a natural blonde. What should I do?

Clairol solemnly advises, "Whatever you do, don't use hair color anywhere except on the hair on your head—definitely not on your eyebrows."

The consultants are telephone psychologists who hear all kinds of other family problems, too.

A caller one day said, "You've got to help me fast. My ex-husband is on his way over here, and he doesn't know I've been getting my hair colored. I don't want him to know I can afford it. I want more alimony. How can I go back to my old color today?"

One woman called to ask whether black was a new color for hair. She went on to announce angrily that her daughter had colored her hair black and looked like a hooker. Then the mother screamed into the phone, "Is that fashionable?"

Some of the most delicate answers are those given to mothers of teenage daughters who try to communicate with their children through the Clairol consultant.

Most mothers find their own hair-color advice unacceptable to their daughters and look to Clairol as the arbitrator in mother-daughter disputes.

Then there are the calls from people who want to dye their hair to match their horse or their dog. Once a man called to see if he could color one spot on his prize heifer. And a woman who phoned in on a July 3 wanted to know if she could color her hair red, white and blue for a party the next day. (She was advised to wave a flag instead.)

Women call, announce their age and want to know if a certain haircut or color is all right for their age. The general advice is that if it makes you feel good, wear it.

Other concerned callers are the first-time blondes. Experience has taught the consultants that the first time a woman goes blonde (particularly if she does it herself at home), she wants to go back to her original color. Often she does, but then the second time she colors herself blonde she never goes back to the darker or drabber shade.

Safety questions come in with great frequency. The most common is—

Will double-process damage my hair?

The answer is that double-process itself is not damaging to the hair because no part of the hair is ever bleached more than one time. The first time the entire head is bleached, and from that time on, only the new growth is touched. Women who color at home are warned to watch overlapping of the bleach because that will weaken the hair and cause breakage.

Also asked is—

How should I take care of colored hair?

The answer is to shampoo, but not too frequently. Clean hair looks best, but it's not necessary to shampoo daily. The hair should be conditioned regularly with an instant conditioner whenever you feel it needs it, and a deep-penetrating conditioner should be used once a month.

What if I want to let my hair grow out?

Go ahead and do it. But first treat yourself to a visit with the best stylist in town. A good cut can always cover a lot of sins.

Ever since the government first questioned the possibility of cancer-causing agents in hair dye, the question of the safety of coloring one's hair has come up off and on. The question asked is—

Will hair color cause cancer?

Clairol states positively that there is no ingredient being used in the manufacture of Clairol hair-coloring products today that can be regarded as a suspected carcinogen. And they add, "Although Clairol products have been reformulated, the company continues to have complete confidence in the safety of the ingredients that were removed."

Each manufacturer issues safety statements, and before using any product, a woman can call or write the manufacturer.

The most difficult inquiries to answer are those that begin, "How do I get my hair a nice blonde color?" The problem is in the word "nice," since one woman's *nice* is another woman's *ugh.*

Celebrities call the number when they need their hair colored for films and plays.

And TV personalities are the ones to whom callers refer all the time. The women callers most want to look like in terms of blondeness are Farrah, Cheryl, Suzanne Somers, Rona Barrett and Dinah Shore.

Now for some other questions consultants deal with.

What's the best kind of product for getting rid of a lot of gray in my hair?

You have choices. You can use a one-step, permanent, shampoo-in hair color for a few gray hairs, but for covering a lot of gray, a creme formula is recommended.

Or use a semi-permanent coloring which covers gray and doesn't change the color of the rest of the hair. To keep your natural look, choose a shade that matches or is slightly lighter than your natural color.

My hair is light, but I'd like to be a definite blonde. Can I do it without double-process blonding?

Yes. Pick one of the permanent shampoo-in hair colors, and go one or two shades lighter than your present color. These products do have the power to lighten your life.

I have light brown hair, and I'm going on vacation. When I come back I want my hair to look as if I've spent a lot of time in the sun. What should I do?

Get one of the special-effects products, because they're gentle and let you control the blonding for the look you want.

Can I mix two colors to get a different shade?

Absolutely! Hairdressers do it all the time, *but you must use the same brand.* Never, ever mix brands.

Do men call the number?

All the time. Their big concern—

How do I cover gray?

Men generally are advised to use a semi-permanent hair color every week.

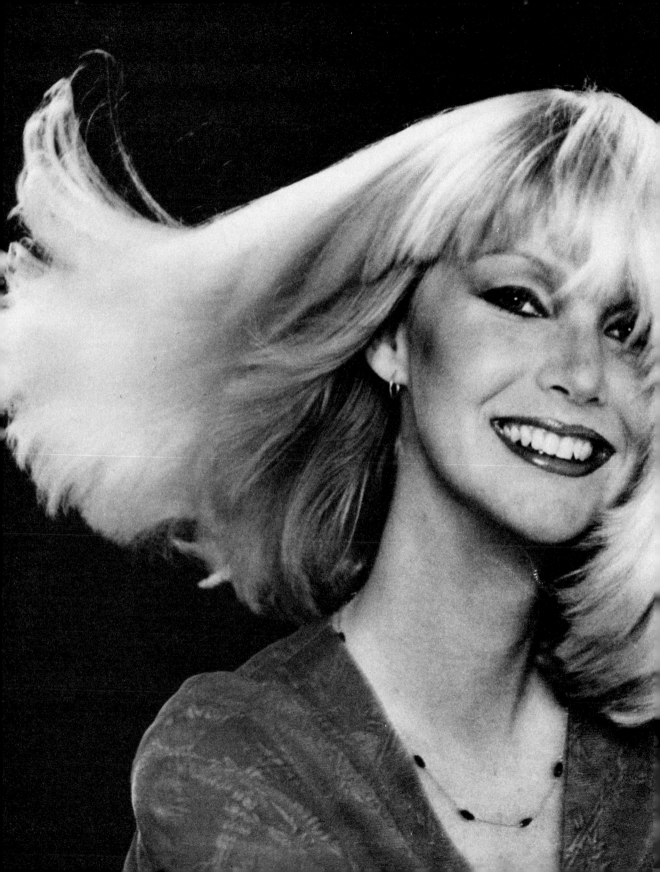

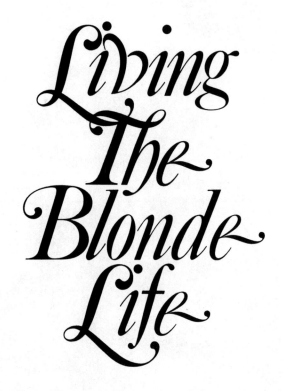

Living The Blonde Life

"If I've only one life . . .
let me live it as a blonde!"

Shirley Polykoff

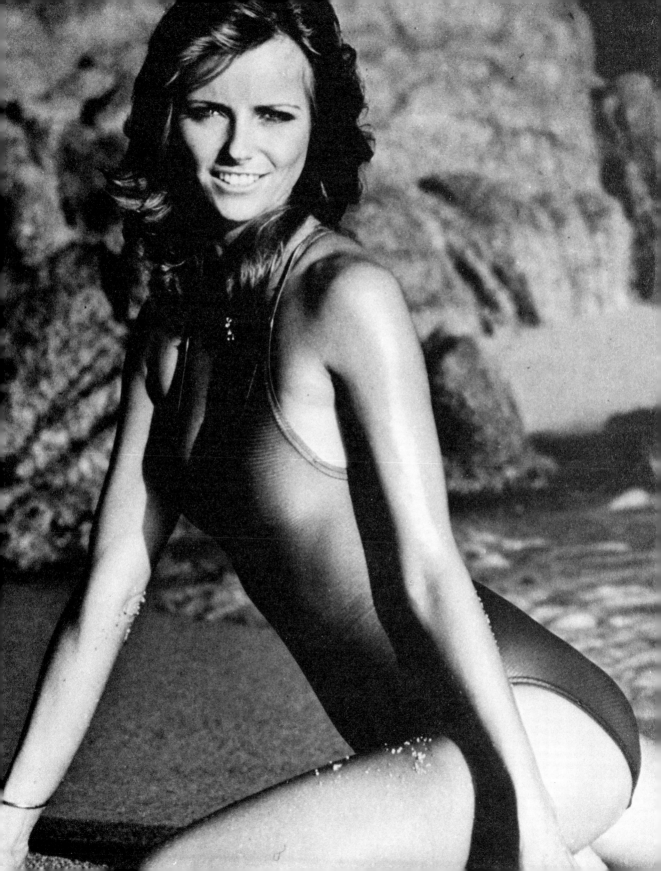

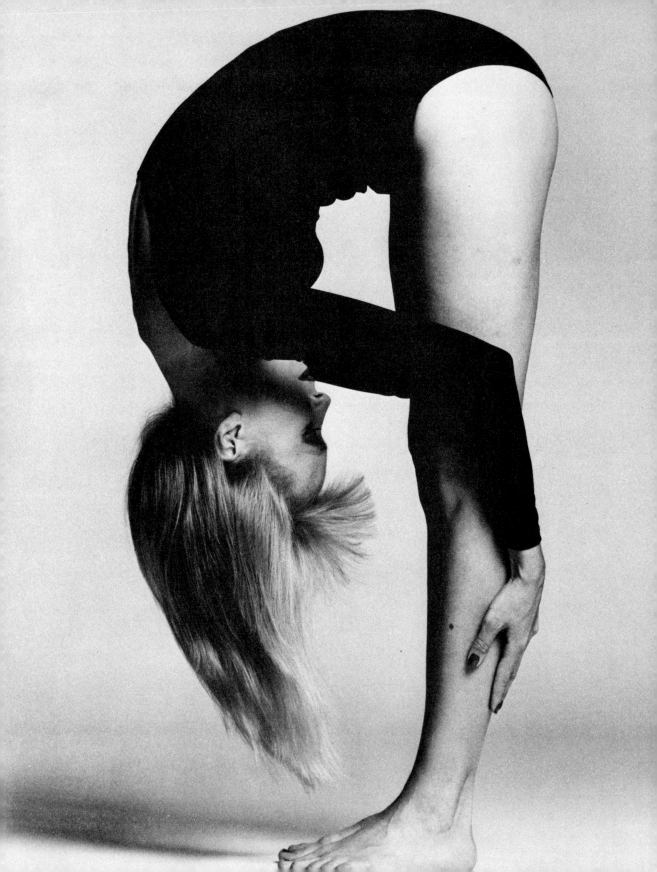

Exercise

"When I was three years old
my mother took me to
Palisades, New Jersey,
where I tried out for
the part of the girl
in the 'Our Gang' series.
I got the part
because I was exactly
what the producers wanted:
a blue-eyed blonde.
And it's always been that way."

Madeline Lee Gilford

In the 1950's advertising copywriter Shirley Polykoff added to The Blonde Myth with memorable lines like "Does she . . . or doesn't she?" and, "Is it true blondes have more fun?"

In the late 1970's Shoi Balaban Dickinson conducted a study entitled "The Meaning of Being Blonde" in which the respondents talked of the pre-1970's image of the blonde as the woman who is more available sexually.

By 1980 most women didn't think that blondeness made them different sexually, but some women interviewed did admit that they thought of the blonde experience as something special.

"I look better as a blonde," one woman said emphatically. "My clothes look better, my skin looks better, and I think women always want to look their best."

Surveys prove that blondes do think about themselves differently. These are some of the things blondes believe:

Blondes really do have more fun.

Blondes feel better about themselves.

Blondes feel more confident just because they are blonde.

Blondes feel softer, more feminine.

Most blondes feel that there really is a blonde kind of body, a blonde way to wear your hair, a blonde way to decorate your home and a blonde way to dress.

Here, then, are the results of the most current thinking on ways to live the blonde life to the fullest.

Of course it takes more than blonde hair to make a blonde appealing.

It also takes a blonde body.

The best blondes are in shape and shapely, and exercise keeps them looking fit.

Which exercises are best for your body?

Depends on which blonde you ask.

Even if she did not supervise the Body Department at Elizabeth Arden, Miss Craig would exercise every day. She believes daily exercise is the only way to help muscles keep their tone. According to this expert, sagging muscles are brought back into shape with exercise, not weight loss. For her own exercise program, Miss Craig concentrates on her abdomen and waist.

Model Christie Brinkley exercises every day no matter which coast she's visiting. In California she jogs two miles on the beach each morning and then swims for twenty minutes. In New York she runs in Central Park, weather permitting, otherwise she opts for a stationary exercise bicycle.

Betsy Palmer, the actress, finds that performing on stage helps keep her body in tone, that the tension and relaxation that's part of bringing a character to life works as a kind of isometric exercise for her.

Dina Merrill, the film star, keeps in shape with sports: tennis, golf, swimming and skiing. And just in case she doesn't have time, weather or equipment for any of those, she climbs stairs.

Now here are some exercise specifics from these four famous blondes.

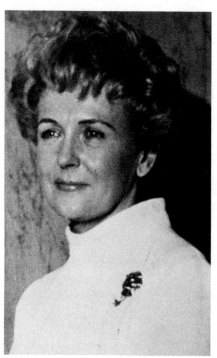

Marjorie Craig

Marjorie Craig's Exercises

To strengthen muscles in pelvis and abdomen:

1. Lie on your back, arms extended on the floor at shoulder level. Palms are up. Bend knees, place feet on the floor close to hips. Feet are together, knees are slightly apart.
2. Keeping your shoulders down, the small of your back on the floor and your ribs up and away from your hip bones, bend your right knee up towards your chest.
3. Raise the right leg and straighten it. Slowly lower the leg to the floor keeping the spine on the floor and the stomach pulled in.
4. Then slowly bend the knee and return the leg to its starting position.
5. Repeat the same movements with your left leg.
6. Do this ten times.

To reduce waist and upper hips:

1. Lie on your back, arms extended out on the floor at shoulder level. The legs are straight and together.
2. Raise the left leg up to the ceiling with the knee slightly bent.
3. Cross the left leg over the body, trying to bring the foot to the floor as close to the right hand as possible. Let both knees bend and the hips roll as the leg crosses over.
4. Bring the leg back up in the air. Straighten it with the knee relaxed and slowly lower the leg to the floor.
5. Repeat with right leg.
6. Do this eight times working your way up to 20 times.

For the abdomen:

1. Lie on your back with your knees bent, feet flat on the floor close to your hips, arms overhead.
2. Sit up and touch your hands to your knees.
3. Return to original position.
4. Repeat ten times.

Christie Brinkley's Exercises

For the thighs:

1. Use a three-pound weight on the right ankle.
2. Lie on the right side, and put the left leg on a chair.
3. Now raise the right leg fifty times.
4. Change sides, and shift the weight to the left ankle.

For the buttocks:

1. Hold the back of a chair for support.
2. Raise the left leg back, bending the right leg slightly.
3. Push the pelvis forward, stretch the left leg as far as possible to the left, and circle bringing the leg back to the original position.
4. Do this twenty times for each leg.

Christie Brinkley poses for a lot of exercise pictures for magazines, is herself a fitness enthusiast, but admits, "I don't always feel like exercising every day, but I force myself to do it because I always feel so much better afterwards.

"I know that if I miss three days of exercise, the muscles begin to lose their tone. Also, I love to eat so I have to exercise. Otherwise I'd be out of a career."

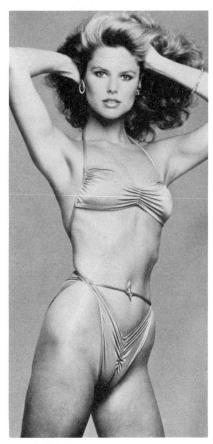

Christie Brinkley
Photography: Francesco Scavullo
Courtesy of *Cosmopolitan* Magazine

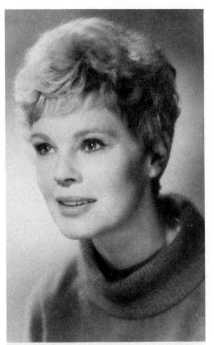

Betsy Palmer

Betsy Palmer's Exercises

Says Ms. Palmer, "Along with my exercise program, I try to maintain a diet of natural foods. I am a vegetarian. I fast one day a week. Eleven days every six months I go on a juice fast consisting of only fruit juices (Dr. Paavo Airola's method).

"I believe fasting cleanses the blood and tissues and effectively regenerates and revitalizes all the body functions."

Betsy Palmer exercises with the MA-roller from The Great Earth Healing Company, Inc. 660 Elm Street, Montpelier, Vermont, because this method stretches the spine.

What is the MA-roller?

It's shaped like a rolling pin with two rounded knobs in the center. The idea is not so much to roll and move, but to rest on the MA-roller and allow it to sink in gently and penetrate every point on your back.

To use the MA-roller:

1. Lie flat on your back and roll it down the top of the head and neck.
2. Lift the buttocks, bend the knees and position it under the shoulder blades.
3. Keeping the buttocks and knees raised, slowly roll it down to the lower back.

How does Betsy Palmer use the MA-roller?

"When you begin you should work with it only a few minutes a day. Gradually you can build up to a forty-five-minute session.

"I also use the MA-roller for my sinuses. I exert slight pressure on the roller as I take it over my forehead and straight down my face to my neck.

"It's slightly painful until you get used to the exercise.

"The rolling action helps keep the spine aligned, and this allows your organs to receive the proper blood supply to maintain your body in good health."

Dina Merrill's Exercises

Dina Merrill works out at the Alex and Walter Physical Fitness Studios in New York, and she's especially partial to the exercises they've developed to help loosen her for skiing.

In addition, Dina Merrill says that she finds occasional body massages help her maintain a relaxed posture and work out muscle kinks, particularly in the neck where tension often settles.

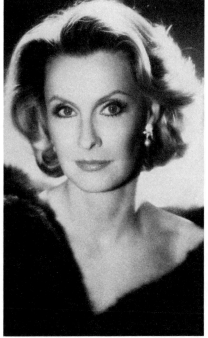

Dina Merrill

To firm thigh muscles and stretch the ligaments and tendons:

1. Stand with feet and toes parallel to each other about three feet apart.
2. Bend both knees and place your hands on them while keeping the back as straight as possible.
3. Move the body from side to side as you press your weight first into one knee and then the other.

To lengthen thigh muscles:

1. Stand with legs about a foot apart.
2. Flex the back foot while keeping it straight and behind you. (Distribute body weight equally to avoid lower back pressure).
3. Place hands on waist and gently bob up and down as you stretch through the back leg. (Let the front leg bend slightly at the knee as you move.)

To relax and stretch the body:

1. Hang from parallel bars and rings.

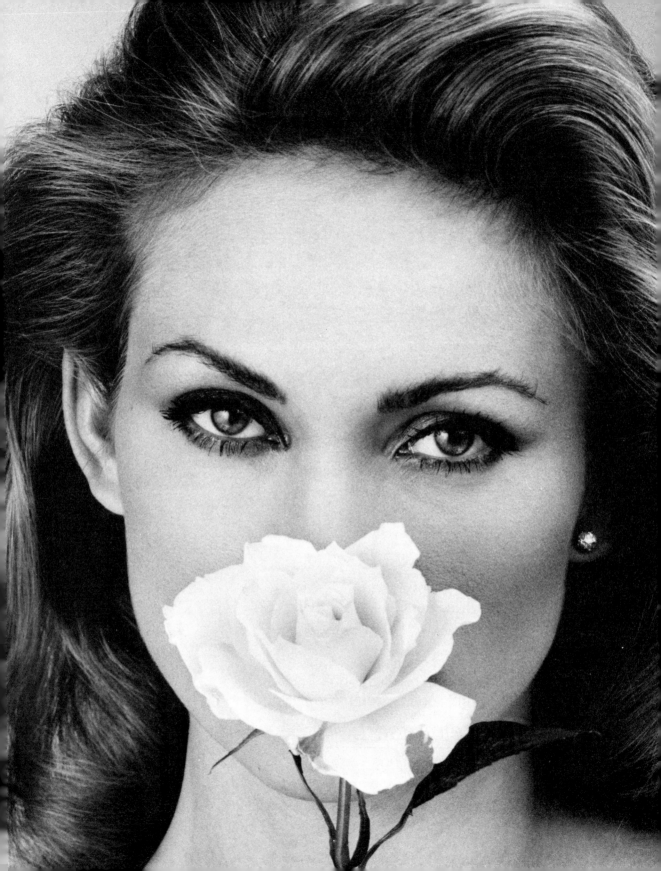

The Blonde Environment

"Most blondes don't really
understand their colors. For instance,
I'll bet every blonde reading this
thinks turquoise is a blonde color.
It's not, you know.
Turquoise comes from South America,
and the only women who
really look spectacular with turquoise
are women who look South American—
brunettes, in other words."

Annelle Warwick
New York/California Interior Designer

What most blondes fail to realize is that the background colors—the places where they work and live—not only set them off to advantage but actually add a dimension to their lives.

The architectural style doesn't matter—nor does the decor. A blonde can look her smashing best in glistening contemporary surroundings, and she can look at home in a country setting.

There is, in fact, no kind of house in which a blonde cannot shine.

All a blonde has to do is decide her philosophy, her life style and furnish accordingly.

The problem is that most blondes tend to reinforce the standard blonde image and make their surroundings both too fragile and too female. Blondes look for yellows and blues for background colors. Or they opt for monochromatic color schemes in grays, pale blues and beige.

What blondes really need is a vivid background. Blondes come alive with room walls in aubergine or brown. (Good backgrounds for your brunette friends, too.) In my own New York apartment there's a lot of beige with a pink cast, a color so subtle that it glows. And it seems to light everyone in the room.

Blondes have to go beyond the boring stereotype of "the blonde room," rooms with a lot of blue or a monochromatic look. What blondes should fear more than bold colors is a bland background, a background that makes blondes a part of the beige color scheme.

It's so much fresher to have instead a red room. Or a deep, dark purple room. Or one with plum tones. If you're a blue-eyed blonde, forget the little girl baby-blue look and make your bedroom lavender—and add lace curtains.

Blondes tend to make more decorating mistakes

than brunettes because blondes err on the side of conservatism. And when blondes reach out to be daring, they often reach in the wrong direction. For example, when zebra rugs were the fashion, blondes used them. Yet it was wrong because that zebra look was definitely a brunette look.

Blondes look best—that is, they look both feminine and fragile—when they are curled up in an oversized chair or cushioned against the plumpness of a big sofa.

Blondes belong in colorful rooms that look like gardens, rooms where a woman can wear high heels, rooms where you can mix antiques with touches of mirrors and tiled or shiny floors.

Blondes are made to sparkle at home in colors that shimmer.

The Look of the Woods: The Scandinavian Blonde

Ideally her home is tucked into the side of a snow-covered mountain surrounded by evergreens. And the look of the woods comes into her home: planked, wood-pegged floors; oversize buttery-soft leather and suede sofas and chairs; a coffee table with a tree-stump base; a pine refectory dining table benched on two sides. She looks best in a large, informal copper-laden kitchen that opens to her spacious dining and living areas. Her bedroom is big and beam-ceilinged, and you reach it by means of a balcony from the living area. All the bedrooms have large, four-poster beds with goose-down quilts. In her bedroom is a fireplace where the smooth-skinned, ski-weary woman can nap on a luxurious fur throw.

A Sense of the Sun: The California Blonde

The interior of her sunny home is decorated in light wood tones. Old oak armoires, tables and chairs are all stripped and bleached. The comfortable and informal sofas are upholstered in colorful cotton prints. And the floors are light hardwood or travertine. The walls are red plum, dark forest green, or deep sea blue—all garden colors—because when you walk through the floor-to-ceiling sliding glass doors you go across a grassy lawn to the swimming pool and/or tennis court.

The kitchen is an important room in her house. The cabinets are all stained in dark wood, and the built-in cooking units are complemented by a high tech restaurant-size range. There is, of course, an indoor spit for barbecuing because even though she can usually grill outdoors, every California blonde has to own every possible kitchen appliance from Cuisinart to microwave oven. The kitchen accessories are rows of copper pans, big wooden spoons and the best cookbook collection on her block.

Expensive and Elegant: The New York Blonde

This woman's sophistication is deceptive. Pale, lovely, willowy, thin and aristocratic, she never looks ostentatious. But she's expensive. Very expensive. She will settle for nothing but the best. Dark polished parquet floors are the background for the finest Oriental rugs; dark lacquered walls provide the background for silk sofas with gleaming Louis XIV tables. What else marks the woman as a New York Blonde? Paul Storer's silver, Staffordshire porcelain, Dresden china, push-button phones, floor-to-ceiling mirrored dressing rooms and baths, dimmers on the lamps, eight down pillows on a king-size bed dressed with imported linen. Plus the caviar and Tab in the fridge.

Cool and Polished: The Palm Beach Blonde

This lucky woman lives like royalty. Well, why not? She's the one who entertains the visiting royalty. She may not dwell in marble halls, but she definitely walks on marble floors. Cool, polished marble floors are one of the marks of her house. The house isn't a house. It's an estate. The rooms have high ceilings and are bordered by 18-foot fan glass double French doors opening onto terraces where lush tropical foliage grows. And it grows perfectly.

There's a terrace extending from the converted ballroom on the north side of the estate to a manicured formal garden with fountains and statuary.

There's no clutter anywhere.

Her house is as unruffled as she.

Modern comfortable sofas are flanked by antique French tables and chairs. A malachite coffee table holds an ancient Chinese cachepot filled with polished pebbles, and tucked in the pebbles is a long limp orchid.

Why does her house run so well?

Because she's personally trained the staff so they know and respect her.

Her gardener admires her knowledge of horticulture.

Her chef is in awe of her gourmet taste.

She's a connoisseur of wine.

And she's at home in Palm Beach.

Antiques and Ancestors:
The Newport Blonde

The Newport Blonde has a home that looks—well, Newport. The house belonged to Grandmama, has all the marks of family living. It's huge, weathered clapboard and stands on a grassy knoll overlooking the sea. The inherited wicker, circa 1906, is sprayed summer white and cushioned in sea blue. The wicker pieces line the veranda that overlooks the croquet lawn. How does the Newport Blonde decorate? She doesn't. Instead of decorating, she's busy repairing. Repairing ancient furniture that is about to fall apart, or has already. Or she may be whitewashing the fireplace in the back parlor, canvas slip covering all existing couches, or repainting the chairs and sleeping sofa. In every room are bold prints and chintz-covered pillows. It's a comfortable, lived-in house run by a lady who's lovely, calm, charitable and charming. Her airy dining room can accommodate sixteen—and often does. Her table always has fresh fruit and vegetables and the catch of the day, which she has fileted herself while standing barefoot in faded jeans and white T-shirt.

Annelle Warwick: in a New York Blonde apartment
Photo: Dick Swift

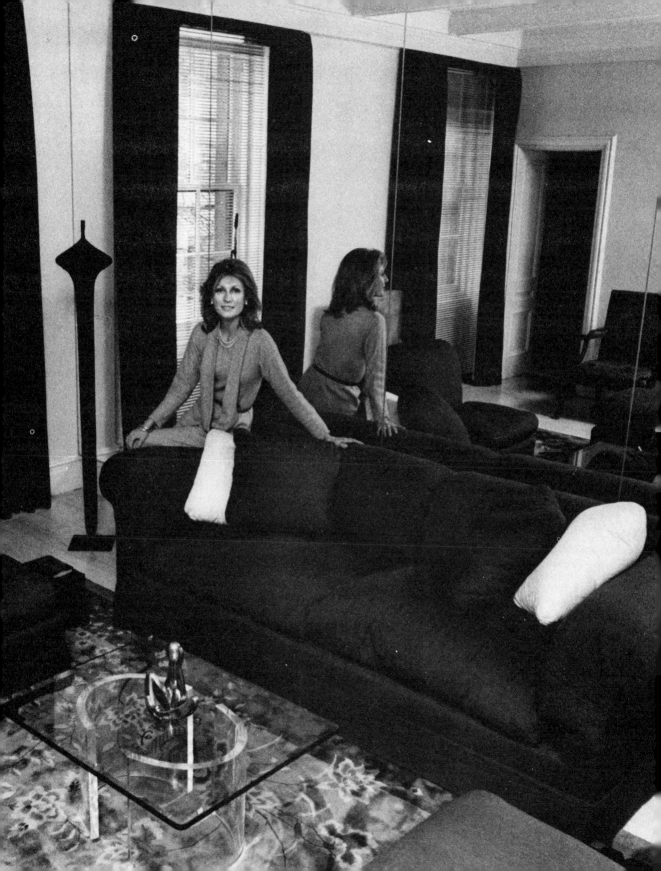

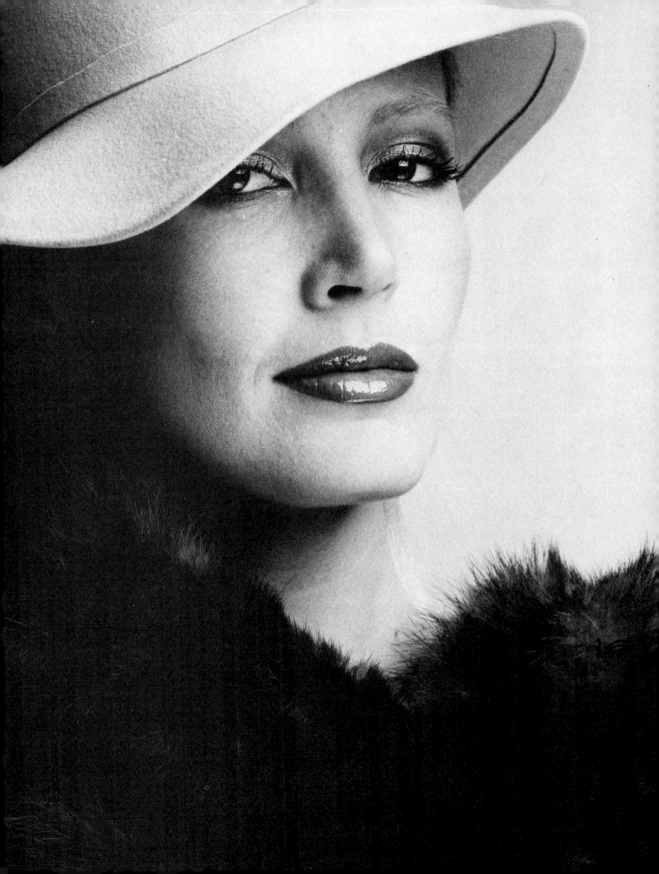

Dressing Blonde

*"In novels, a heroine is always blonde—
if not in her head, then in her soul.
After all, gold is only the treasure
a hero seeks—while a true heroine
is the treasure he finds."*

Lois Gould

There's just one fashion rule: Know your look and stay with it. Take the time to discover and develop your style, and then don't change it with the seasons or from day to night or at any other time. If you're a tailored woman by day, don't turn into a soft and ruffly bunny at night. Your own person can't handle that.

Blondeness is like a terrific accessory. Your hair and your coloring are the focus. Everybody else is looking for a focal point: blondes begin with one.

But even though the look should stay the same, colors can change. Emily Cho, the author of *Looking Terrific,* likes the no-color colors for blondes: beige, bone, white, taupe, greige. She calls them "the classics."

"All women dress for a good response," says Cho. "There are fabrics that help a woman understand herself. For instance, if you are a pale and fragile blonde and want more presence, start wearing fabrics with more body. Instead of limp ruffles, wear silk shirts or soft wools, challis. And if you feel too masculine, it can be to your advantage to wear less rugged clothes. Leave the tweeds and gabardines in the closet, and look for softer lines and fabrics."

Cho likes to work with blonde clients. She describes them as "a clean palette" and against that palette she can apply any texture and color.

Giorgio Sant'Angelo thinks nighttime color can do a lot for a blonde. Sant'Angelo, the designer whose night clothes light up the best parties around the world, loves blondes in black, red or blues. But, like Annelle Warwick, he cautions, "Any blue except turquoise."

And he takes exception with Cho; he eschews beige. "Blondes look washed out in beige," he says. "And blondes shouldn't get near yellow. They're good in green, especially bluish greens." He also likes dusty colors for blondes: dusty pink, blue and gray. "But no one in America understands gray," he moans.

Sant'Angelo thinks blondes can discover their best

colors with a simple trick. He says, "Find a blouse that matches the color of the blonde in your hair. Then see what colors go with that blouse. The colors that work best with the blouse will work best for you."

What's the best look for each style blonde?

The Scandinavian Blonde looks wonderful in rough-textured clothes, rugged sweaters, jeans. At night her best look is the understated sheath, the kind Halston does so well. Colors? Black is spectacular.

The California Blonde has the most pulled-together look of all. She can wear any of the classics, and she has the presence to mix extremes. For instance, she can wear a huge jacket and skinny pants, or jeans with high-heeled sexy sandals. At night the soft look of silk jersey pants and tops.

The New York Blonde has a tendency to look too perfect, too matched, too trendy. She should surprise her audience with an offbeat touch. Instead of wearing one designer slavishly, she needs to mix designers, should work at adding her own thoughts to her costumed look. Generally, the New York Blonde looks as if she's trying too hard, is never relaxed. She has to work at communicating a less aggressive attitude. At night she'll look less pre-packaged in a silk shirt and soft skirt—the perfect restaurant outfit.

The Palm Beach Blonde with her perennial tan is the one blonde who can wear bright colors all year round and all around the clock. Vibrant-colored halter-neck and strapless long dresses look at home in the flora and fauna that surrounds a Palm Beach Blonde.

And as for *The Newport Blonde,* well, she's so secure she can still wear her Papagallos, T-shirts and Lilys. Her nighttime look is a longer view of the day look: long plaid skirts, sweaters, frilled white blouses. She doesn't even have to try for a good response. It's just there. She's non-threatening, and women love her. So do men.

The thing to remember is that you can bend all the rules, and even break a few, as long as you can stand in front of a mirror and say, "I'm glad I'm me."

Furs

Blondes don't just *wear* furs; they make a *statement* about them.

A blonde makes a fur a part of her personality, an extension of her looks, remembering always to let her blondeness be the focal point. The most successful blondes create their own environment, and while a blonde doesn't have to feel beautiful all the time, she certainly has to when she wears fur.

The Scandinavian Blonde should match her own natural wild look in furs like long-haired coyote, tanuki or fox.

California Blondes (especially if they live in California) want lightweight furs designed for the active life. Their best bets are high shades of mink or beaver, particularly some of the new ribbed looks.

New York Blondes emphasize their sophistication when they wear sable, fisher or dark mink.

The Palm Beach Blonde should underscore her own subtle elegance with lynx, cat lynx, Russian lynx or any other spotted furs.

The Newport Blonde can wear her mother's inherited mink or her college beaver coat. It looks fine, as does her camel-colored cloth coat.

Jewelry

If you still think of diamonds and Lorelei Lee whenever you hear "blonde and jewels," take another look.

Even though Zsa Zsa Gabor is never without a pair

of diamond earrings, she says, "I have lovely emeralds, rubies, sapphires, but I think there is nothing better than a nice plain necklace and accessories of blue-white diamonds."

Pat Tuck of De Beers Diamonds Ltd. notes, however, that most diamonds have a little tinge of color and suggests that blondes look good in a diamond with a tinge of yellow, the one often called a canary diamond. And, in case your friends should ask, you might tell them that the Tiffany Diamond is one of those.

Luca Buccellati, jeweler to the rich and famous, likes emeralds set in yellow gold for the blonde woman. He also suggests rubies, but finds diamonds and sapphires less beautiful on a blonde.

Says Buccellati, "Blondes should wear warm metal, yellow gold. I like it better than silver or platinum, but in a formal piece certainly platinum is appropriate."

Yellow gold, he notes, is very much in vogue these days and has been used at Buccellati for generations.

In today's society, blondes and jewels have changed.

The Scandinavian Blonde: Her jewelry is as simple and unaffected as she. Around her neck is a little chain with a diamond in the middle, and diamond studs glitter in her ears (her ears are pierced, of course).

The California Blonde is never seen without her Rolex oyster watch. She must wear a waterproof, shockproof watch (always in anticipation of the Big Wave), and just above the watch on the same wrist is her Cartier chain. Around her neck is a gold chain with an offbeat pendant. She wears a grouping of narrow rings on two or more fingers or one super pinkie ring.

The New York Blonde wears at least one gold bracelet always and has a diamonds-by-the-yard choker, an everyday big no-stone chunky ring, and at least one big pin which may be sprinkled with diamonds. She keeps time with a Santos or a Cartier Tank watch (the real one, not the copy) and wears a chain around her neck (but heavier than the Scandinavian Blonde's).

The Palm Beach Blonde is a David Webb customer and has a real feeling for gold with diamonds. Neck, ears, lapel—she's got the right David Webb piece. But on her wrist is Corum's gold ingot watch.

The Newport Blonde wears the jewelry that's been in her family for generations—or no jewelry at all. Her watch is by Timex. After all, she can afford to be thrifty.

Glasses

Glasses are as much a fashion accessory as earrings.

What kinds of glasses work best on blondes?

For sun and sports wear, try rose-tone lenses with rose frames. Avoid blue or gray lens colors; they tend to dull blonde looks.

If you have a small face, wear a rectangular frame.

Larger faces require larger frames.

And an elongated face should never wear too-small glasses. Be certain the frames come lower on the cheekbone.

The right glasses can help compensate for the wrong features.

Today the smart blonde shops for her eyeglasses as carefully as her clothes. An eye examination and a pair of eyeglasses can cost over $100 or under $50.

Big, tinted lenses are always more expensive and more likely to carry such designer names as Christian Dior, Givenchy, Diane Von Furstenberg, or Oscar de la Renta.

For my money they really are better designed than the ordinary no-name glasses. And they're worth the big price tag as much as a good belt or handbag.

The Do's and Don'ts of Beautiful Blonde Dressing

• Do wear black, lots and lots of black.

• Do keep your clothes simple; avoid the wild swings of fashion.

• Do remember that of all the things you can wear, nothing is more important to your looks than that head of blonde hair.

• Do make your clothes less important than your total look.

• Do find a piece of jewelry, wear it all the time and make it part of your signature. (It can be a string of pearls, a gold bracelet, a chunky ring.)

• Do wear scarves, chokers, earrings—anything that keeps the eye up toward your blonde hair.

• Don't fall in love with a very expensive high-color dress, shirt or suit. You won't be able to wear it often because the color drains your blonde look.

• Don't wear combs in your hair, earrings and a choker at the same time. Remember, in framing your face, as in everything in life, less is more.

• Don't use a lot of color in your wardrobe. Instead do a basic look for yourself in black, another in beige, and use color for accents.

• Don't wear flat shoes all the time; blondes look leggier and sexier in high heels and stockings.

• Don't spend all your money on the big stuff; save some so you can have a rotating wardrobe of scarves, belts and shirts.

• Don't think that underwear doesn't matter. Even if you're not planning to get hit by a bus, it's important to feel like a woman and wear lace under the tweeds and gabardines.

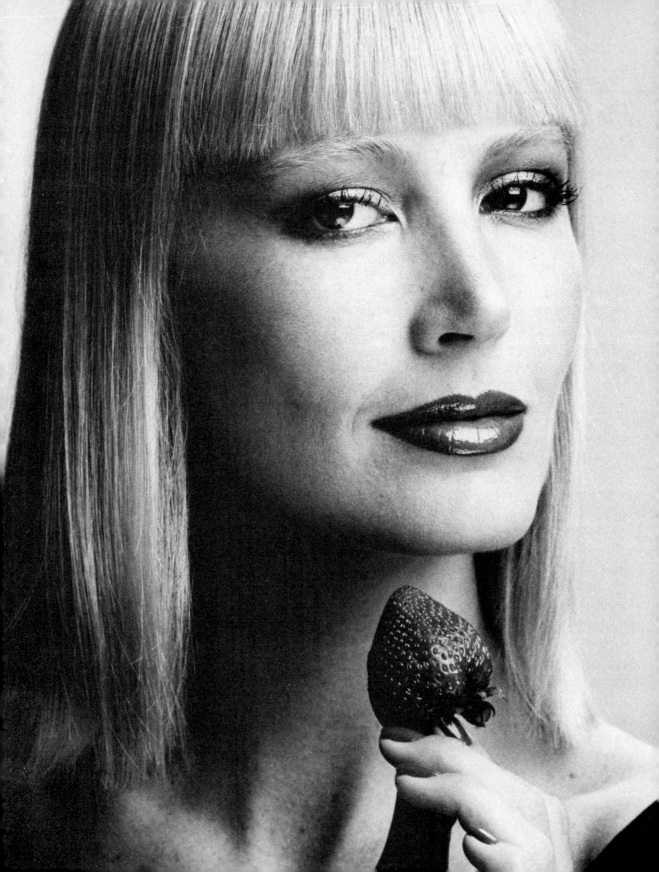

The Care & Feeding of Blondes

*"When you start eating
for healthy hair,
the improvement should come
in about six months.
It takes at least six months
of proper eating
before you can see
any real improvement in your hair.
But if you pamper it and feed it,
well, your blonde halo
will indeed be your crowning glory."*

Lois L. Lindauer

In nineteenth-century literature we had the image of the pale, fragile blonde. She was the heroine dying of consumption, the wasp-waisted lady under the parasol.

Today that fragile look is no more.

And we are also beyond the antithesis of that look, the natural (meaning no makeup) look of the 1960's and 1970's.

Now, in the 1980's, women are headed toward a new kind of prettiness—a kind of good looks that is based on health.

This is the era of healthy body, healthy mind, healthy looks.

As a result of this new standard of looks in women, you need more than a hair color that flatters. You also need a body that's in tune with our times.

As we've all been told, the right body begins with the right nutrition.

Lois L. Lindauer, who is International Director of the Diet Workshop, a group that works with individuals and groups to promote healthy living, is convinced that good nutrition is the most important factor in all health, including the good health of the hair.

She points out that beauty and nutrition experts may disagree on specific foods that promote healthy hair, but that most agree protein and the vitamins B complex and E are necessary for healthy hair.

Since protein is not stored in the body, it must be eaten daily (and hair is 97 percent protein, in case you wondered how important protein is).

The Foods Your Body Needs

Meat, fish, poultry and eggs are excellent sources of protein. At least one beauty expert swears by eggs. Mary Ann Crenshaw, author of *The Natural Way to*

Super Beauty, says that if your doctor finds your cholesterol level low, "you're free to discover the egg and its wonderful effect on hair."

Gaylord Hauser notes that the Chinese people in general have thick, luxuriant hair that keeps its color until late in life. Their diet—soybeans, soy sauce and a great variety of quick-cooked vegetables—is rich in the B vitamins. They also eat sea greens which contain iodine, and that's important for healthy hair, too, as is the fish and seafood consumed by many Chinese.

Lois Lindauer recommends other good sources of B complex including wheat germ, brewer's yeast, black-strap molasses, nuts, cheese, milk products and leafy green vegetables.

She points out that wheat germ is a good source of vitamin E, and that helps keep hair from becoming dry and dull—and falling out. Other good sources are dark green vegetables, eggs, liver, oil and organ meats. Vegetable oil is low in cholesterol and does help give a sheen to your hair—but oh, does it have calories!

Liver, a good source of two of the "healthy-hair vitamins" A and E, can be made in interesting and new ways. (Included in the recipe section is a unique liver recipe, "Liver à la Bali.")

Blonde and Shapely

Leslie Blanchard, the hair colorist, says, "A woman can't just color her hair and expect to be a sexy, gorgeous woman. You can't get it all from a bottle."

So while healthy comes first, shapely is a close second. Getting to your ideal body measurements through proper eating is what this section is about.

Lois Lindauer has developed a special diet designed to improve your body quickly (take off weight fast) and then maintain and continue the weight loss.

The Blonde Blitz-It-Off Diet: A Fourteen-Day Plan

Want to blitz it off with a diet?

Here are the facts about this fourteen-day diet:

• You can lose seven to twelve pounds in two weeks.

• Expected weight loss is four to seven pounds the first week, three to five pounds the second week.

• Eat three meals a day at regular times.

• Snack only as indicated.

• Make no food substitution.

• Weigh all protein.

• Measure the vegetables.

• Broil all chicken and fish.

• Drink as much coffee and tea as you wish (no milk or cream).

• Drink diet beverages at any time.

Breakfast

¼ cup orange or grapefruit juice or ½ cup berries
  and
1 egg or 2 ounces cottage cheese
  and
1 ounce pumpernickel, rye or wheat bread
  and
coffee, tea, decaffeinated coffee or diet beverage

No one should skip breakfast.

If you work (or rush around getting breakfast ready for a family), prepare your own breakfast the night before. Leave your juice and cottage cheese in the fridge—ready for you to eat and run. Have your slice of bread in the toaster and water ready to boil.

Of course you could get up 15 minutes early and do all this in a leisurely fashion. But whatever your method, don't skip breakfast and think you can eat more at a later meal.

Dieting doesn't work that way.

Lunch

3 ounces clams, cod, flounder, haddock, sole, scallops, shrimp, water-packed tuna or chicken
and
Green salad with 1 tablespoon diet dressing
and
1 ounce pumpernickel, rye or wheat bread
and
¼ honeydew melon or ¼ pineapple or ½ cup berries or ½ cup juice-packed pineapple
and
Coffee, tea, decaffeinated coffee or diet beverage

This lunch is designed so you can eat easily in a restaurant or at home (or at your desk if necessary— but about that, more later).

The important thing is to *count.* The amount you eat is as important as what you eat.

Dinner

6 ounces fish or 4 ounces of chicken or turkey
and
½ cup cabbage, mushrooms, lettuce, spinach or zucchini (just one, please)
and
Fruit (choose from that luncheon list)
and
Coffee, tea, decaffeinated coffee or diet beverage

Does it matter in what order you eat the foods?

No. Some women prefer to start with fruit because the sweetness tends to curb the appetite. Others prefer that sweetness at the end of the meal.

If you want a before-going-to-bed snack, try:

1 glass of skim milk or six ounces of plain yogurt (I've found that if you add two spoonfuls of instant decaffeinated coffee and some liquid sweetener to plain yogurt it makes a good-tasting bedtime dessert.)

Keeping It Off

Anybody can stay on any diet for two weeks. (After all, we've all done it six or seven times each year.)

But how do you keep it all off?

Lois Lindauer says resolutely that there's just one trick: *Stay within the calorie range your body can burn weekly.*

How do you find it?

Here's how to figure.

First, for the approximate number of calories your body burns each day, multiply your ideal weight by 12. That means if you want to weigh 110 pounds, your body should burn 1,320 calories a day.

Multiply that figure by seven to determine how many calories your body should burn weekly. For the 110-pound woman, the figure is 9,240.

Find your number, and don't exceed that number per week.

What's the advantage of maintaining weight this way?

It means you can save for a sunny day. Hoard a few calories here, a few calories there, and get set for a wild weekend.

The Wild Weekend

If weekday eating isn't important but those eating-out weekends are, here's the plan for you.

Consume 1,200 calories daily Monday-Friday.

If you're that 110-pound woman, you've "saved" 120 calories each day. And you have the weekend to spend the extra 600!

Here's another way to figure for yourself.

If you consume 1,200 calories daily for five days, you've used 6,000 calories. Now subtract 6,000 from your weekly allotment—and what fun you can have!

The Working Woman's Maintenance Plan

Whether you work or stay home, this much is true: A nutritionally balanced diet for all women includes foods from the four basic groups *every day:*

Protein (meat, fish or poultry)

Dairy products

Fruits and vegetables

Grains (breads and cereals)

And even if you can't get to a restaurant (and work outside your home), there's a way to keep lunch nutritional and within your calorie safety standards.

We've included some great recipes for brown-bagging but first here are a few extra tips for the working woman who is eating in.

- For meat sandwiches, use sliced chicken, veal or turkey in place of luncheon meat.
- For dessert, pack an apple, an orange or other fresh fruit in season. No cakes, pies or cookies.
- An open-face sandwich, sealed in plastic food wrap, gives you half the bread, is twice as smart.

Comes the day when the meeting goes on and on, you look at your watch and someone says, "Let's call the deli for sandwiches."

How do you stay diet-safe with a deli?
- Order à la carte: Those plate specials are loaded with hidden calories.
- Sliced chicken and sliced turkey are best bets.
- Number One Summertime Choice: Cottage cheese with melon.
- Specify thin-sliced bread if you order a sandwich.
- If they insist on sending a roll, eat only half.
- Don't touch the mayonnaise: Use mustard instead.
- Order a tossed salad dry, and use the small pack of low-cal dressing you keep in your desk or handbag for such emergencies.
- Hungry? Really hungry? Then fill up on pickles. Dill or kosher style have only eight calories each.

The At-Home Maintenance Plan

As a mother who has spent many noon hours standing at the sink finishing what's been left in the refrigerator, I know the problems (another word for temptations) of eating at home.

The best way to watch at-home eating is to watch at-home shopping and cooking. Here are some hints:
- Make a thorough inspection of your kitchen shelves and get rid of all the highly processed mixes and food extenders (they're loaded with calories).
- When you sauté, use bouillon or tomato juice, not butter or oil.
- Use pan spray or lined pans rather than cook in butter, margarine or shortening.
- Start putting fish, poultry and veal on the weekly menu and wheel your cart right past the pork, ham

and beef.
- Broil, don't fry.
- Trim all fat before cooking meat.
- Flavor vegetables, soups and meats with lemon, herbs and spices instead of butter or salt.

Does this mean you can never have good-tasting dinners at home?

Of course not.

Lois Lindauer has some Diet Workshop recipes for the blonde you on the following pages.

Eating Out

You go to a friend's home for dinner, and she serves everything you know is going to get you back six pounds. What to do?

Don't embarrass her. Don't make a fuss. Just push the food around the plate, nibble enough to be sociable, and make up for this at the next meal.

But when you go to a restaurant, the choice is generally yours. So here's the best way to order and maintain your weight.

Instead of liquor, start with a glass of white wine or a white-wine spritzer (white wine with soda) or bottled water. The wine has from 50 to 90 calories.

For your entrée, stay with your basics: broiled fish, seafood or poultry.

Vegetables: string beans or zucchini.

Order your salad dry, and use lemon or vinegar. If there's a salad bar, go easy. Stay with the greens. No croutons. No chick peas (¼ cup contains 180 calories). Bacon bits? Only if you know that one tablespoonful adds as much as 30 calories to your dinner.

For dessert? The old faithful. Fruit.

Unless, of course, this is your wild weekend. Then you figure it out, you smart blonde.

The Delicious Blonde Diet Recipes

The following recipes were created and tested by Lois L. Lindauer for *Blonde Beautiful Blonde.*

Blonde Blitz-It-Off Recipes

Bored by the sameness of dieting?

Try these recipes, a new one for breakfast, one for luncheon and one for dinner.

Breakfast Blitz: French Toast

2 slices Melba Thin Dietslice Bread
1 egg, well beaten
Sweet 'n Low to taste
cinnamon

1. Soak bread in mixture of egg and Sweet 'n Low.
2. Sprinkle with cinnamon and broil each side until brown. Yummy.

Luncheon Blitz: Tuna Sandwich on Toast

1½ ounces water-packed tuna
¼ cup cottage cheese
1 teaspoon horseradish
2 slices Melba Thin Dietslice Bread, toasted
thick wedge of lettuce

1. Mash tuna, cheese and horseradish together and spread on toast.
2. Top with lettuce for a mile-high sandwich.

Dinner Blitz: Velvet Chicken Tandoori

8 ounces plain yogurt
2 teaspoons ground coriander
1 teaspoon curry powder
½ teaspoon salt
⅛ teaspoon pepper
dash Tabasco
2 tablespoons vinegar
2½ pounds chicken pieces (broiler-fryer), skinned, with all fat removed

1. Combine yogurt, seasonings and vinegar to make a marinade. Prick chicken pieces with fork and make cuts into thicker areas to aid marination process. Cover chicken completely with sauce and let stand in refrigerator for a full day or overnight; the longer the chicken is marinated, the spicier it will be.
2. Arrange chicken in baking dish, cover with marinade and bake at 350 degrees for 45 minutes or until tender.
Serves 4.

Brown-Bag Recipes for the Working Woman

Chicken Salad

2 cups diced cooked chicken
1 cup celery sliced diagonally
¼ cup dietetic French dressing
¼ teaspoon green onion salt
2 tablespoons lemon juice

To make this elegantly delicious chicken salad, simply toss all the ingredients together and pack in a plastic container.
Serves 4.

Tossed Salad

Make your tossed salad with mixed greens, cucumber rounds, green pepper and purple onion rings. Pack in a plastic container that doubles as a salad bowl at your desk.

Yogurt Dressing

3 cups plain yogurt
1 teaspoon parsley
¼ teaspoon garlic powder
¼ teaspoon onion powder
dash salt and pepper

Mix together with wire whisk or spoon. Refrigerate in a small jar that you can take to the office. Mix a tablespoon with your tossed salad and save the rest for future use.

Pineapple Fluff

1½ envelopes unflavored gelatin
3 cups liquid skim milk
3 packets Sweet 'n Low
2 teaspoon pineapple extract

Sprinkle gelatin on cold milk in saucepan. Cook over low heat until dissolved. Add sweetener and extract. Chill until syrupy. Beat at high speed until fluffy and double in volume. Spoon ⅓ of recipe into a container to travel. Serves 3.

Even without facilities for refrigeration, you can still have an interesting, tasty and low-calorie brown-bag lunch at your desk. Try this:

Salmon salad sandwich mixed with Thousand Island dressing
Celery, carrot and cucumber sticks
Jelly roll
Tea with lemon and Sweet 'n Low

Salmon Salad Sandwich

2½ ounces canned salmon
chopped green pepper
1 tablespoon prepared low-calorie Thousand Island dressing

Mix salmon, pepper and dressing. Spread on diet slice bread, top with lettuce.

Jelly Roll

2 eggs, separated
1 tablespoon water
1 tablespoon vanilla
¾ cup Alba non-fat dry milk powder
¼ teaspoon salt
¾ teaspoon cream of tartar
½ teaspoon baking soda
5 packets Sweet 'n Low

Combine egg yolks, water and vanilla. Add milk powder and mix until smooth. Beat egg whites until foamy; add salt, cream of tartar, baking soda and sweetener while still beating, and beat until stiff. Fold egg whites into powdered milk mixture. Spread in 7" x 11" non-stick sprayed pan. Bake in 350 degree oven for about 8 minutes. Remove from pan and roll up with sheet of wax paper inside roll. Cool. Unroll. Remove wax paper. Spread with thin layer of dietetic jam and roll up. Wrap a slice in foil for traveling.

Create your own brown-bag lunches. Experiment with leftovers or new ideas. Here's a tip:

Tuna salad makes a nutritious lunch. Instead of mayonnaise, mix with cottage cheese, tomato juice, dietetic salad dressing, crushed water-packed pineapple, mustard, horseradish or pickle juice. Pack in a plastic container and it's ready to commute to work.

Maintenance Menu Makers

Remember.

Maintenance dining doesn't have to be boring. Here are some recipes that add to your reputation as a good cook—and a thin cook.

Spinach Quiche

1 package frozen chopped spinach, thawed and drained
1 tablespoon celery, chopped
1 tablespoon onion, chopped
½ cup mushrooms, sliced
1 tablespoon parsley flakes
6 ounces Swiss or Gruyère cheese, sliced paper thin
2 eggs, lightly beaten
1½ cups evaporated skim milk
1 tablespoon flour (optional, and for maintainers only)
¼ teaspoon white pepper
dash salt
¼ teaspoon nutmeg

1. Combine spinach, celery, onion, mushrooms and parsley flakes. Spread on bottom of Teflon pie plate or quiche pan. Cover with slices of cheese.
2. Combine eggs, milk, flour (if being used) and seasonings. Mix well. Pour mixture over spinach and cheese. Bake at 400 degrees for 30 minutes, or until a toothpick inserted near edge comes out clean. Serve as an appetizer or main dish.
   Serves 4.

Party Swedish Meatballs

1 cube beef bouillon
½ cup hot water
3 tablespoons minced onion flakes
12 Melba Rounds, garlic or onion flavor, blended into crumbs
½ cup evaporated skim milk
1½ pounds very lean hamburger, ground fine
¼ pound veal, ground fine
1 egg, lightly beaten
¼ teaspoon salt
½ teaspoon freshly ground pepper

1. Dissolve bouillon cube in hot water. Sauté onion flakes in broth.
2. In a large bowl, soak crumbs in milk; add sautéed onions and remaining ingredients. Mix thoroughly.
3. Shape mixture into small balls, wetting hands to keep mixture from sticking. Broil meatballs on rack on flat pan for about 15 minutes, turning once or twice. Remove to a chafing dish. Pour sauce over meatballs (recipe below). Serve hot.
Serves 8 as appetizer.

Sauce for Meatballs

½ cup pan drippings
½ cup evaporated skim milk
pepper to taste

1. Stir milk into pan juices gradually over low heat. Simmer 2 to 3 minutes, stirring occasionally. Add pepper. Pour sauce over meatballs.

Beef Stroganoff

1½ pounds round or flank steak, very lean
salt and freshly ground pepper to taste
1 cup sliced mushrooms
1 medium onion, chopped
2 cloves garlic, minced
1½ cups beef bouillon
1½ teaspoons prepared mustard
½ teaspoon garlic powder
½ cup cottage cheese, blended smooth (or 5 tablespoons sour cream—for maintainers only)

1. Remove all fat from steak. Broil steak medium rare. Cool.
2. Cut steak into thin strips about 2 inches long and 1 inch wide. Season the strips with salt and pepper. Refrigerate one hour.
3. Sauté mushrooms, onions, garlic and meat in ¾ cup beef bouillon till browned. Discard the garlic.
4. Heat ¾ cup bouillon in saucepan. Add mustard, garlic powder and cottage cheese. Stir over medium-high heat till blended. Pour sauce over meat and simmer for 3 to 5 minutes.
Serves 4.

Eating Well Is The Best Revenge

When they turn to you and say, "Oh, you probably starve all the time," you can truthfully say you've never eaten better.

Because when you count calories, watch your foods, it's true. Nutritionally you're sound. And you'll find being thin and comfortable in your own body is the best way to live.

But that doesn't mean you can't eat excellent food.

Here are some recipes to add to your culinary reputation.

Liver à la Bali

1 teaspoon dried onion flakes
1 teaspoon garlic powder
¼ cup vegetable bouillon
1 packet Sweet 'n Low
⅛ teaspoon black pepper
½ teaspoon crushed red pepper
½ teaspoon salt
1 bay leaf
½ cup tomato juice
1 pound calves liver, sliced
2 tablespoons soy sauce

In skillet, mix together all ingredients but the liver. Cook a few minutes until boiling. Lower heat, add liver and cook about 5 minutes until liver is tender.
Serves 2.

Polynesian Stir-Fry Shrimp

½ teaspoon seasoned salt
⅛ teaspoon ginger
½ teaspoon onion powder
½ teaspoon garlic powder or 1 clove garlic, crushed
½ cup water
1 tablespoon lemon juice
2 cups celery with leaves, chopped
3 green peppers, cut into strips
1 pound shrimp, cleaned, uncooked
1 cup pineapple chunks packed in own juice, drained

1. Combine seasonings, garlic, water and lemon juice. Marinate shrimp in mixture for one hour.
2. Spray pan with non-stick spray and set at medium-high heat (325 degrees on electric fry pan).
3. Stir-fry celery and green peppers, using small amounts of marinade liquid.
4. Add shrimp, stir until cooked, about 5 minutes.
5. Add drained pineapple and simmer 2 minutes, stirring gently. Serve piping hot.
Serves 2.

Chicken Hawaiian

16 ounces boned chicken breast, cut into chunks
1 teaspoon paprika
dash Tabasco sauce
1 tablespoon lemon juice
1 packet Sweet 'n Low
2 cloves garlic, minced
1 tablespoon minced onion flakes, softened in water
¼ cup orange juice
½ cup frozen chopped spinach, partially thawed
½ cup carrots, sliced on the diagonal
½ cup canned mushrooms, sliced
½ cup onions, sliced
¾ cup diet pineapple chunks packed in own juice, drained
ground pepper to taste
½ medium cabbage, shredded

1. Sprinkle chicken chunks with paprika, Tabasco, lemon juice and sweetener and toss well.
2. Spray heated skillet or wok with non-stick pan spray.
3. Stir-fry garlic and onion flakes in orange juice.
4. Add all vegetables to pan, stir-fry 2 minutes.
5. Add chicken and spice mixture and stir till chicken is cooked—about 5 to 7 minutes. If more liquid is needed, add ¼ to ½ cup water.
6. Add pineapple and simmer for a minute. Add ground pepper to taste. Serve on bed of shredded cabbage.
Serves 4.

Teriyaki Steak

1 four-ounce can tomato sauce
1 tablespoon soy sauce
½ teaspoon garlic powder
minced garlic to taste
¼ teaspoon ginger (optional)
1 tablespoon minced onion flakes
1 four-ounce can sliced mushrooms or 1 cup fresh mushrooms, sliced
3 dashes Worcestershire sauce
¼ cup water
pepper to taste
1 tablespoon vinegar
1 pound flank steak (London Broil)

1. Mix together all ingredients except steak.
2. Slice steak into thin strips, cutting on the diagonal, then cut the slices into 2-inch pieces.
3. Marinate steak in mixture for 2 hours, turning pieces a few times.
4. Using stir-fry cooking method, cook at medium-high heat for 3 to 5 minutes or until steak is done. Garnish with scallion flowers.
Serves 2.

NEW YORK TIMES, WEDNESDAY, NOVEMBER 28,

Counter Quotations

TUESDAY, NOVEMBER 27,

The Executive Blonde & Other Power Blondes

*"I consider myself completely feminine,
even if I am in a man's world.
It would be very good for women
to remain completely feminine
no matter what business they are in.
They can get away with murder!"*

Eva Gabor

Ever since Mary Wells Lawrence burst onto the American business scene and became the highest-paid woman executive, blonde has been a bonus in the boardrooms of America.

Power blondes are everywhere. Their Gucci/Bottega Veneta/Hermès bags and briefcases are their trademark; Caleche and Chamade, their scent; Calvin Klein, their high priest of daytime dressing; Mary McFadden, Saint Laurent and Chloe, their designers by night.

In the Power Blonde's briefcase you'll find blusher, eye shadow, mascara as well as books, papers, magazines, a small umbrella and a cotton kerchief for her hair (never silk—silk slips; cotton holds).

She owns The Basic Raincoat—a beige trench coat—and probably has at least two others. One travels with her at all times.

Her wardrobe includes silk shirts, slim skirts and plenty of suits, jackets and low-key clothes to set off her high-voltage look.

Sally Jessy Raphael

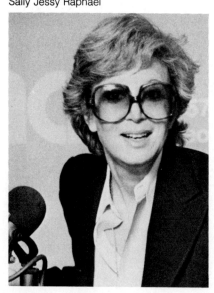

A blonde viewer of the blonde power scene, Sally Jessy Raphael sees major differences between blondes and brunettes. Sally has her own radio show in New York and runs one of New York's trendy East Side restaurants, The Wine Press.

"Blondes have the advantage every time," Raphael says with authority. "A smart blonde can't be beat. She's a study in contrasts. If she's high-powered, tough and strong in business, then she wears her blonde hair fluffy. She wears silk shirts, soft clothes. That's what appeal is all about anyway: contrast. I have a shy friend, and she wears her hair in a severe style and has only tailored clothes. That kind of dressing gives her confidence. A power blonde doesn't need that.

"The real secret is that people expect less of these glamorous women, so they are able to accomplish more."

As a restaurateur-cum-interviewer, Sally has put together her own blonde philosophy. It's part of the world of Blonde vs. Brunette.

Sally is quick to admit that she doesn't dislike brunettes; it's just that she thinks blondes are better. Outrageously better.

"Blondes live, think and act better than brunettes," says Sally. And here is some of the evidence she cites.

Brunettes are the ones on the six o'clock news, and they're all named Judy. Blondes are the ones who produce the six o'clock news.

For brunettes it's all over at 30. A good blonde can go to 50.

Brunettes wear boots all year round; blondes wear strappy sandals.

Brunettes eat baked potatoes in foil, carrots and spaghetti sauce with meatballs, and they cut up their steak into little pieces and take it home in a doggy bag where they eat it alone. Blondes eat pasta primavera, lobster, country paté and black bean soup with Madeira, and they order a big steak and eat it all at the restaurant with a marvelous man.

Brunettes always want to get married; blondes want to have fun.

Brunettes collect Impressionists; blondes want Rembrandts.

Brunettes display pottery; blondes have porcelain.

Brunettes wear granny gowns; blondes go to bed in lavender and lace.

Brunettes ski in Pennsylvania; blondes go to Gstaad, Sun Valley and Sugarbush.

Brunettes marry football players who run corporations. Blondes run the world.

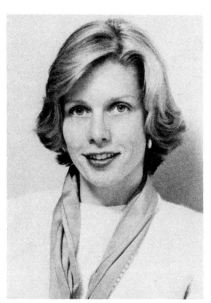
Cathi Black

Cathleen Black is another kind of power blonde. After graduating from college in 1966, she came to New York and went to work as an advertising salesperson for Curtis Publishing Company. Today she's the youngest (and only woman) publisher of a general-interest magazine. Her magazine is *New York,* and her style is New York.

"Back in 1972," Cathi Black recalls, "women like me were careful to be very businesslike. We all knew we were in the forefront of women who did things, so even though a lot of women in those days were beginning to wear trousers to the office, I was one of those who overcompensated. I wore skirts and blouses and suits.

"As an executive now it's all different. I'm more comfortable about myself. I can wear more feminine clothes to work. I used to stick to browns and beiges and maroons. Now I wear brighter colors—purple, black, white, mauve, red."

Does being blonde make a difference?

"Absolutely. All my life I've felt better, special because I'm blonde. I really like it. In high school I was afraid I wasn't blonde enough, so I colored my hair. Now I don't do anything drastic—just a little highlighting a couple of times a year."

Cathi Black is convinced people look longer, harder and with more interest at blondes. "I used to have a brunette roommate," she recalled, "and even though she was prettier than I, when we walked down the street people looked at me first."

In her office Cathi Black doesn't want to make a statement. She prefers a comfortable office with few things around to distract her, a working environment. Her office colors, unlike her wardrobe, are terra cotta and beige.

But she's convinced clothes and office all contribute to the aura of blonde. Is it important to be blonde?

"Of course," she says emphatically. "Did you ever hear of a brunette described by her hair color? Nobody says 'the brunette publisher.' But they all say 'the blonde publisher.' "

If you called Central Casting and asked for an executive blonde, they'd probably send Suzan Couch. She's got everything going for her: brains, looks, breeding and a first-class job. She's a vice-president at American Express and travels all over the world in her job.

Suzan was born blonde, has been blonde all her life except for a slight lapse in the 1960's when she decided to be natural. "I was gray for about a minute and a half. It was awful, absolutely awful," she says with a small shudder.

"I thought being blonde took too much time, but during that ninety seconds when I was gray I learned that how you feel is more important than saving four hours every quarter."

Suzan Couch lives every minute of her life remembering she's a blonde. Her favorite place in the world is her beach house where the walls are white, the wood is bleached white and even the bare wood floors are painted white and polyurethaned to a high gloss. "I do have one blue wall with that Chagall poster of Nice, the one with the mermaid. Everything else is glass and light. It looks like the south of France, but it's in the Hamptons so it's a lot easier to get to from the office."

A sunshine person, Suzan's convinced that all blondes look best in the sun. Where, in the whole world, does this American Express executive think blondes look best?

First choice is Hôtel du Cap at Cap d'Antibes because "the awnings and canvases in that sensational blue color are perfect for blondes in the sunshine."

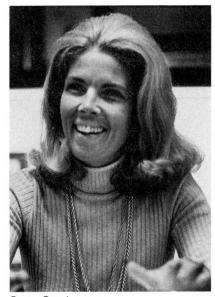

Suzan Couch
Photo: Maje Waldo

Second is Rome, anywhere in Rome, because Italian men tend to think blonde women are patrician and wonderful. And, she notes, Italian men like you anyway just because you're female. Another bonus in Rome is the pale gray velvet background of the restaurants and the abundance of flowers on the table. For absolute perfection in a blonde's Roman life, there should be a suite at the Hassler. The mauve color does a lot for romance.

Third place for a blonde is a spa. Take your choice. It can be a spartan place like Maine Chance or a sybaritic one like La Costa. "Personally I'll take La Costa," says Suzan Couch. "When you go there you can cheat a little, and in between all that good, healthy stuff you can go off to the fish restaurant for a little Dom Perignon and lobster."

Next choice for a great blonde background is any dark boardroom. If a dark boardroom isn't available, Suzan Couch recommends a light boardroom. "Nothing," she said with a small, secret smile, "absolutely nothing does more for a woman's looks than a boardroom."

How does the executive blonde pack for a business trip?

There are two schools of thought: the Pack Everything School and the Pack As Little As Possible School. Halston believes that a woman should be able to go anywhere in the world on 24-hour notice and be able to pack everything she needs in one bag. In that bag Halston would put: a raincoat (one that's fur-lined with removable lining), a soft dress, a pant suit, a blouse and skirt, a cardigan sweater that goes over everything, walking shoes, dress shoes, a cosmetic bag which also includes soap, wash cloths, instant cleaning packets (for refreshing oneself when soap and water are not available) and cleansing tissues. Halston also recommends one outfit to wear for parties or the theater. And when packing he advises to stick to a single color. His suggestions: black or beige. To spice it, use scarves and colorful shirts. The traveling blonde's jewelry should include a gold chain or chains, a wristwatch, gold earrings, pearls and pearl earrings.

Personally I subscribe to the Black Skirt School of Packing.

I go everywhere in the world with two pieces of carry-on luggage. I wear a suit, carry a hanging bag for two black skirts—one for day, one for evening—a variety of blouses and sweaters, one dress, jeans and a jacket. The only jewelry I take is pearls and a gold chain. And I tuck at least three books in the bottom of the bag.

I also carry a squashy bag, and that has all the other things I need: makeup, lingerie and et ceteras.

I save all the sample sizes that you get at department store cosmetics counters and use them for travel. I also take a hair drier, shampoo, conditioner—and a lightweight electric steamer, a small iron that steams out all the wrinkles in seconds (a trick I learned from model sessions). I wear an all-purpose coat, take three belts and carry four scarves: one big enough to serve as an evening wrap, one for my head when it rains and two as accessories for those black sweaters. And I always pack three pairs of shoes: one low-heeled daytime, one high-heeled daytime and one evening. I also take one small flat bag for evening use.

How long can I stay with this kind of packing?

Two weeks.

Suzan Couch believes in living the full, rich blonde life wherever you are. She rarely travels light, always overpacks. "Everybody tells you to trim down, leave things at home. Wrong. I say, 'Take everything. When in doubt, pack it.' "

Among the things Suzan packs: a fur coat and a trench coat. (Never leave the fur at home, she advises.) She will pack as many as twelve blouses, all on hangers to avoid pressing and the problem of finding hangers in hotel closets. "There's no hotel in the world with enough hangers, pillows or towels," she said. "When I walk into a hotel room, I pick up the phone, call housekeeping and immediately ask for more. You don't even have to look. You can be sure there won't be enough hangers, pillows or towels."

To keep her blonde looks when she travels, Suzan has hot rollers and driers in all currents. "The adapters never seem to work," she said knowingly. "Always take 220- and 110-volt appliances with you. I can't tell you how many times I've bribed a hotel electrician to come in the middle of the night and change the adapters for me."

When she travels (with American Express she's always on the move), Suzan Couch shampoos her own hair. She also shampoos her own hair during a regular work week. "My best times are Sunday and Wednesday, Sunday when I come in from the beach at five in the afternoon, and Wednesday, either in the evening or at 5:30 in the morning." Her hair takes her 45 minutes to an hour from shampoo to finish.

Her beauty regimen is a shampooing followed by a good heavy conditioner. Then she blows her hair almost dry, puts in hot rollers to set and blows the rollered hair dry at 1200 watts for ten minutes. "I have thick, strong hair so it works. I don't know if that's the answer for fragile hair," she admits.

As more women come into the office, sexual awareness has taken on political overtones.

Sexual-harassment suits are cropping up among unlikely old-line companies and involve new-style women.

Are more blondes sexually harassed than brunettes?

There are no statistics, but there are opinions.

Kathy Keeton, the glamorous blonde associate publisher of *Penthouse* and *Omni,* has her own ideas about sexual harassment.

"There's no such thing as sexual harassment if a woman watches the way she acts. In my own case," confides Ms. Keeton, "I try to look sensual and sexy and act like a lady. I always visualize a glass wall between myself and a man I'm doing business with. I never give a man the opportunity to make a pass because then I'd be forced to refuse, and I'd lose a friend.

"My own formula for seeing men is: lunch, fine; drink, fine; but no dinner out unless there's another person in attendance. I think a woman can make it very clear at an early stage that she likes, respects and admires a man—and that's it.

"Men make super friends," says Keeton, "and the more male friendships you have, the better off you are in the business.

"But," she says with a shrug of her shoulder, "don't lead men on."

Kathy Keeton

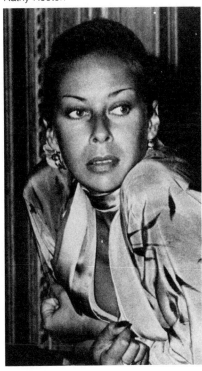

The Network Blondes

By the late 1950's women had begun to infiltrate the all-male ranks of television news. Their role? Weather girl. Betsy Palmer was one of them on the "Today Show." By the end of the decade there were 42 weather girls on TV stations throughout the United States—and 40 were blonde.

The "girls" have moved up in the last 20 years. Now they're women, and they're rarely the weather reporters. Instead they're delivering hard news and tough opinions.

On NBC the morning begins with Jane Pauley on the "Today Show." At the same hour on CBS is Leslie Stahl, and on ABC we get Joan Lunden.

Throughout the day and evening more blondes deliver more news. There's Catherine Mackin on ABC, and on NBC Jessica Savitch as well as Pia Lindstrom (the daughter of a classic blonde, Ingrid Bergman). On ABC Pat Collins is one of the resident blondes.

So what does that mean?

Is that what the trend to light news signifies?

Beth Trachtenberg, a blonde producer, takes an impartial view. "It's easy to figure. Blondes tend to be less threatening. Tell me, when was the last time you met a sultry blonde?"

Trachtenberg's view is that women sitting at home won't feel inferior to a blonde.

Which may or may not be good news.

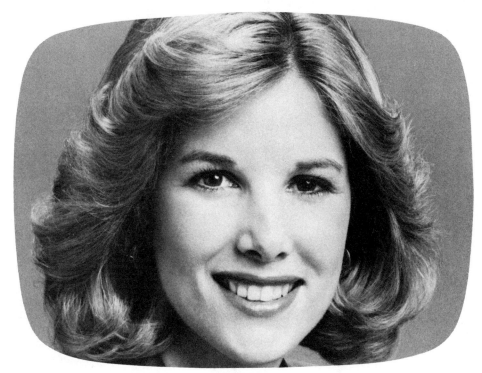

Joan Lunden

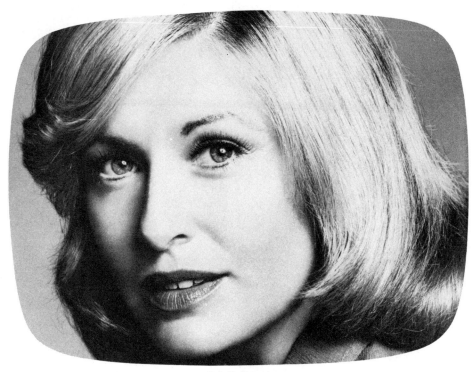

Pat Collins

167

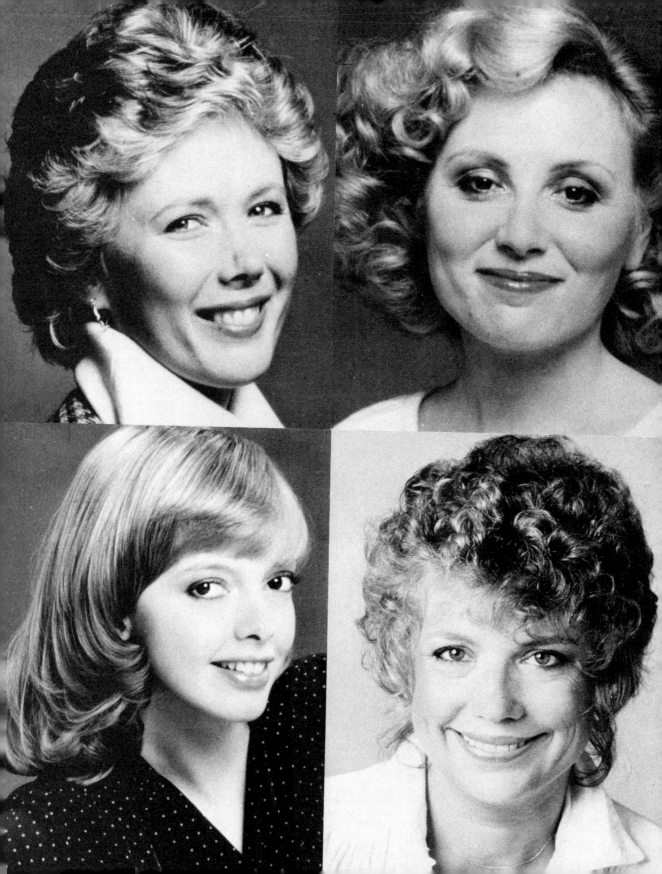

The Rewards of Blonde

"In the seventh and eighth grade the girls really don't sense any difference between blonde and brunette, but by the ninth grade it's very important. The brunettes are all turning blonde— with a little help from their friends."

*Julianne Schick,
Teacher at the Andrews School
Willoughby, Ohio*

Blonde has become the symbolic key to unlocking the full sexual potential of a woman. In some cases, of course, this is more than the woman can handle. The classic example is Marilyn Monroe, who was turned from a brown-haired woman into the sexual fantasy of every male. And Marilyn Monroe found that it was easy to be the secret mistress of every man. What was difficult was being the real-life love of one man.

Recent studies have shown that there's more to blonding than sexual fulfillment.

Dr. Judith Waters, professor of psychology at Fairleigh Dickinson University, conducted a research study to find whether improvements in hair color, hair style and makeup could increase a woman's salary potential. What the study proved is that it does pay to look one's best.

Dr. Waters took a group of women between the ages of 25 and 55, photographed them as they came into the studio and then photographed them again after the makeovers.

The "before" photos were taken as the women really appeared. No one tried to make the women look less attractive; no harsh lighting was used, nor were any of the women asked to remove makeup, change their hair style or otherwise alter their appearance.

After the first photography session, each woman was given a haircut, had her hair colored, and had makeup designed for her face. Then she was re-photographed.

The "before" and "after" pictures were then attached to each woman's résumé and presented to personnel managers of large companies and agencies that employ women of varying backgrounds. The résumés and photographs were rotated so that all photographs and résumés were shown in combination an equal number of times. Each potential employer was shown three photograph/résumé combinations, but never "before" and "after" photographs for the same job applicant. They were asked to rate each applicant and estimate how much she could expect to earn.

The study showed that women applying for entry level jobs could earn from 8 percent to 20 percent more money simply by improving their appearance. As Dr. Waters remarked, "It takes a lot longer to improve skills, and while all of us recognize that basic skills are important, we cannot overlook the significance of a woman's good grooming."

Here are some of the makeovers:

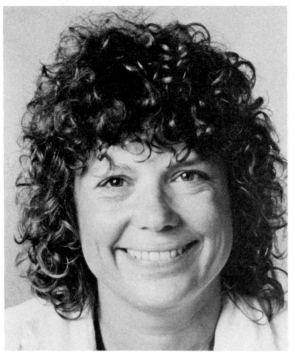

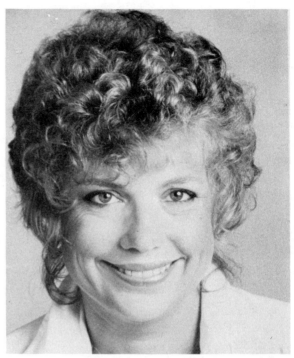

Carole

Before

After

Carole went from dull blonde to glamorous golden with a shampoo-in hair coloring. And her "after" salary estimate went from dull to glamorous golden, too; it was an increase of 12%. In Carole's case the short haircut set off the new color to its best advantage.

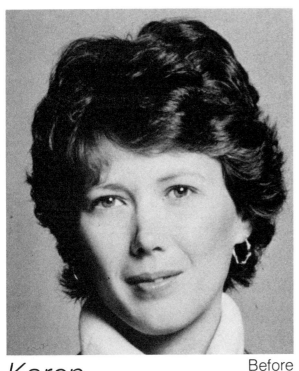

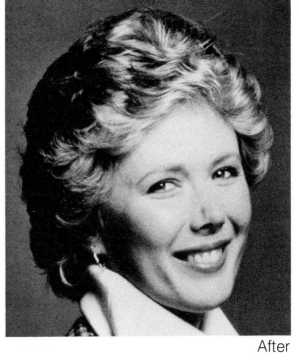

Karen

Before

After

Karen not only increased her salary potential as a blonde, she increased her confidence. Because she didn't want a lot of fuss and bother with her hair, she chose frosting and colors her hair only three or four times a year. But she loves the change and says, "I feel good about myself."

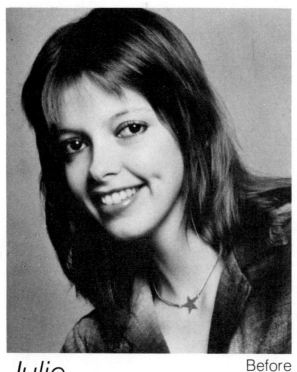

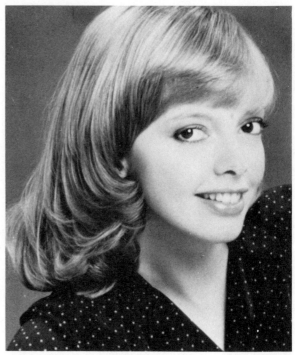

Julie

Before   After

Although she looks attractive as a brunette, she looked ever more employable
as a blonde. Julie's hair was lightened
several shades with a shampoo-in formula, and because color gave her hair
more body, it also made it easier to man-
age; she looked neater and more efficient.

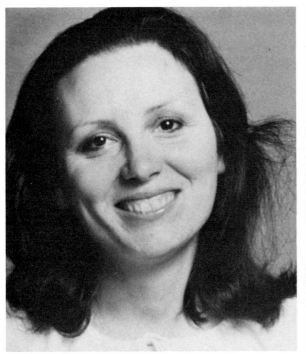

Sylvia

Before

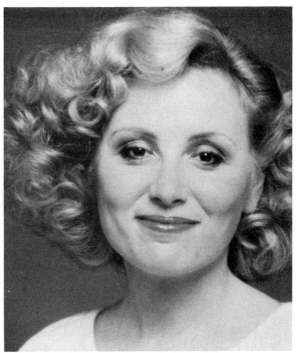

After

An actress, Sylvia wanted a part in an important play, but the role was written for a blonde. In order to get a blonde look, Sylvia went to two-step blonding. She did get the part, and she did stay blonde because she decided that's the way she really liked herself.

When brainy women like Nancy Kissinger (she now wears blonde streaks) go lighter, it's a signal that more than sexuality is involved in blonding. It's the personal reward of looking one's best.

And now Dr. Waters has given evidence of still another reason. "The social advantages of attractiveness have long been documented," she reported. "This was the first study done of the effect in dollars and cents of looking good in the work situation, and it boils down to a question of self-image. The implication is if she cares about herself, she probably relates better to others. It may not be fair to judge a person's capability by her appearance but the results indicated that (either consciously or unconsciously) employers definitely do."

This study should be of greatest significance to the older woman returning to the work force. She's the woman who needs most to have her confidence boosted. When she knows she looks her best, she will be more confident, and that shows when she's talking to potential employers. That's especially true for blondes.

Blondeness is the fastest, least expensive way for women to return to the work force with self-assurance.

And it's the way for women of all ages and life styles to increase their confidence.

Of course no woman wants to be noticed, rewarded or loved solely for the color of her hair. William Butler Yeats once wrote these words:

For Anne Gregory

Never shall a young man,
Thrown into despair
By those great honey-coloured
Ramparts at your ear,
Love you for yourself alone
And not your yellow hair.

But I can get a hair-dye
And set such colour there,
Brown, or black, or carrot,
That young men in despair
May love me for myself alone
And not my yellow hair.

I heard an old religious man
But yesternight declare
That he had found a text to prove
That only God, my dear,
Could love you for yourself alone
And not your yellow hair.

The Last Word

I never expected to write a book about blondes.

I write novels, and I write poetry, and I once wrote a book about what it's like to be the wife of a very successful man. Beauty books are really slightly off my typewritten path.

But when Linda Exman suggested the book, I jumped at the chance to write it. And now that it's done, I can sit back and wonder just what made me agree so quickly.

All I can honestly say is that I've been absorbed by The Blonde Myth all my life, and instinctively I wanted to find out why. Did it begin in the kindergarten with my best friend Julianne Purvis, and my coveting her blonde looks? Was the myth intensified by adorable blonde high school cheerleaders like Betty Arthur and Eileen O'Donnell? Was it hyped by the pure and total and secretly desired sexiness of Marilyn Monroe?

Now that I can think in leisure, I guess it's all of these things and none of them. I became blonde long after any of those women was a conscious influence. I became blonde because I was ready for change—and blonde was available, affordable and non-threatening. Now I find that what blonde has really done for me is postpone the middle years. My children are grown, yet I still feel I'm growing up. Blonde makes me feel young and good and ready to tackle the world.

No, I know blonde isn't about to replace intelligence, warmth, humor and womanliness. I'm still working on all those things from the inside.

Blonde has given me a kind of confidence that typing sixty words a minute never did.

I know I don't have to be blonde to be successful in business.

But being blonde makes it more fun.

I'm glad we're beyond the days when everyone assumed that homely girls were smart, and pretty girls were born dopey. I think it's smart to be pretty. And I guess what I like best about all the research done for this book and all the things I've learned is that now we can prove that it even pays to look good.

I've raised my children in a world where ugliness stars on the six o'clock news. I walk to work on city streets that are piled with garbage and debris. I live near a park you can't enter at night because only God knows what goes on in its confines. And that's just the man-made ugliness.

I'm sick of ugly.

I've always believed that women were put on earth to add beauty. And even though I think we have to endure a lot of ugliness, I still think it's a woman's role to make the world look better.

And why not begin with ourselves?

I don't think it's silly, wasteful and extravagant to spend time and money improving your looks.

I think it's downright unfair—to yourself and the people you live with—not to look as good as you can.

And I haven't found anything that works faster, better or makes you feel more beautiful than being blonde.